The Miracle of
VEGETABLES

The Miracle of
VEGETABLES

The Scientific Facts About Nutritional Properties and Medicinal Values of Vegetables

Dr. Bahram Tadayyon

To order additional copies of this book, contact:
Xlibris Corporation
1-800-618-969
www.Xlibris.com.au
Orders@Xlibris.com.au
503288

CONTENTS

DEDICATION

To my parents, Mohamed Taqi Tadayyon and Fatima Kal-Awadh, who from early childhood infused in me the importance of education and supported me from fifty-seven years ago to embark on the pursuit of knowledge wherever that might be.

Any five servings of vegetables a day will keep doctors away.

(Dr Bahram Tadayyon)

INTRODUCTION

Hippocrates, the father of Western medicine, said, 'Let our food be our medicine, and let our medicine be our food.'

Recent epidemiological research has shown that vegetarians live longer than non-vegetarians and lead a life of better quality, with less chronic diseases.

The word vegetable is derived from Latin *vegetabilis* (animated) and *vegetates* (active) referring to the plant growing.

Vegetarian is the person who, for either health reasons or humanitarian cause, does not eat meat or other animal derivatives like eggs and dairy products.

Vegetable can be a whole plant or part of a plant, such as root, stem, leaf, flower, bulb, fruit, or seed.

The application of the word 'vegetable' is somewhat arbitrary, based on culture; for instance, in some cultures, potato is considered to be a cereal like rice and mushrooms are considered vegetables although they are not plants.

Nuts, grains, herbs, and spices are not considered as vegetables.

The plant parts used as vegetables are as follows:

- Roots: beets, radish, rutabaga, turnip, horseradish, jicama, sweet potato, parsnip, cassava, carrot, daikon
- Leaves: Swiss chard, spinach, cabbage, kale, collard, lettuce, parsley, Brussels sprouts, endive, arugula, bok choy
- Flower: broccoli, cauliflower,
- Stem: bamboo shoots, kohlrabi, asparagus
- Tuber: potato, sweet potato, yam, Jerusalem artichoke

- Bulb: onion, garlic, chives, shallots
- Corm: taro, water chestnut
- Rhizome: ginger
- Leaf sheath (petiole): rhubarb, celery
- Entire plant: khainam (water eggs)
- Seeds: corn, beans, peas
- Buds: Brussels sprouts
- Stems of leaves: celery, rhubarb, cardoon
- Whole-plant sprouts: soybean, alfalfa

Fruits used as vegetables: tomato, cucumber, squash, pumpkin, bell peppers, eggplant, okra, beans, peas, corn. They are technically fruits because they develop from the ovary of a flower and they contain seeds that develop from ovules inside the ovary.

Vegetables can be divided into starchy, fibrous, and leafy types.

Starchy vegetables include beans, beets, carrot, cassava, corn, pea, potato, sweet potato, pumpkin, rutabaga, squash, taro, turnips, and yam. They contain complex carbohydrates, which satisfy appetite and curb desire for sugars. They have medium to high glycemic index, which is more than that in fibrous and leafy vegetables. Nutritional value of starchy vegetables is not necessarily less than the other groups; for instance, carrots are rich in carotenoids and beets have high content of anthocyanins. To avoid gaining weight or increasing blood sugar in diabetics, the daily intake of this group should be limited to one serving only.

Fibrous vegetables include alfalfa sprouts, artichoke, cauliflower, broccoli, chard, lettuce, celery, spinach, cabbage, eggplant, kale, rhubarb, mushrooms, onion, and bell peppers. As the name implies, this group is very rich in dietary fibres.

Leafy vegetables include more than 1,000 species of plants with edible leaves, such as lettuce, spinach, cabbage, bok choy, molokhia, and arugula. This group is rich in vitamin K, vitamin C, folic acid, carotenoids, iron, calcium, and magnesium.

Vegetables are eaten in a variety of ways as main meal, salads, soups, snacks (celery sticks, carrot sticks, and cherry tomato), juice (tomato, carrot, and veggie), and desserts in pies and cakes (pumpkin, carrot and rhubarb).

Vegetables can be eaten raw, canned, frozen, juiced and dried.

Vegetables can be steamed, cooked, stewed, sautéed, fried, grilled, and poached.

We need at least five servings of vegetables per day. Most people do not get even two servings. Go for a variety of types, textures, and colours to obtain maximum benefit because there is not one vegetable that supplies all the nutrients. Every vegetable offers unique flavour, aroma, texture, and nutritional value. Dark green vegetables (like spinach) have chlorophyll, yellow/orange vegetables (like carrot) contain carotenoids, red vegetables (like tomato) contain lycopene, and purple vegetables (like eggplant) contain anthocyanins.

Serving size of vegetables is based on the portion size that people normally eat, ease of use, and nutritional content. The amount of one serving for different types of vegetables is as follows: cooked or raw vegetable is half a cup, leafy raw vegetable like spinach and lettuce is one cup, vegetable juice is half a cup, vegetable-derived products like ketchup or tomato paste is half a cup, tomato is one, corn is one ear, broccoli floret is five, baby carrot or celery stick is ten, pea is nine, French fries is ten, and onion is four slices.

HEALTH BENEFITS OF VEGETABLES

Daily consumption of vegetables can lower the risk of many diseases, improve overall health, and rid the body of harmful substances. Each vegetable has its own unique nutritional values and medicinal benefits but in general,

1. Vegetables are low in calories and fat but are rich in fibre, vitamins, minerals, and flavonoid antioxidants, and some contain proteins and/or omega fatty acids.
2. Vegetables are ideal to include in weight management programmes. Some vegetables are starchy and caloric-dense and hence are excellent to increase weight in undernourished individuals. Some other vegetables are non-starchy and are composed mainly of water and fibre and are ideal to include in dieting programmes.
3. Medicinal vegetables like onion and garlic have antibiotic properties.
4. Some vegetables like Swiss chard, radish, and turnip help in detoxification of carcinogens and toxic substances.
5. Some vegetables lower blood pressure, cholesterol, heart diseases, and stroke.
6. Certain vegetables protect against some types of cancers.
7. Some vegetables are diuretic and rid the body of excess fluids and waste products.
8. Most vegetables are rich in fibre, which absorbs excess water in colon and helps smooth passage of faecal matter out of the body.
9. Most vegetables are rich in vitamins C and A and phytochemicals, which boost immunity.
10. Some vegetables are rich in sugar and thus boost energy and help overcome fatigue.
11. Some vegetables prevent night blindness and delay the onset of cataract and macular degeneration.

12. Some vegetables are rich in iron, copper, and vitamin C that aid in red blood cell formation and prevention of anaemia.

13. Some vegetables contain calcium, phosphorus, magnesium, zinc, and vitamin K, which work synergistically to build strong bones and prevent osteoporosis.

14. Some vegetables are rich in folic acid and prevent neural tube defects in newborn infants if consumed by pregnant women.

15. Some vegetables prevent nervous system disorders like Alzheimer's disease, insomnia, and depression.

16. Some vegetables prevent menstrual and/or postmenopausal symptoms.

17. Some vegetables have anti-inflammatory properties and relieve arthritic pain and lower the severity of asthma.

18. Many vegetables have anti-ageing properties and keep hair, nail, and skin healthy.

19. Most vegetables keep the body alkaline and thus aid in maintaining a high state of overall health.

20. Many vegetables are fat burning. They increase metabolism, converting energy from foods into the energy needed to perform the necessary functions.

GO ORGANIC

It is a common knowledge now that organic vegetables are superior to the traditional varieties because organically grown vegetables never use pesticides, synthetic fertilisers, sewage sledge, genetically modified organisms, and ionising radiation. Pesticides are linked to neurotoxicity, immune suppression, and disruption of endocrine system, decreased reproductive function, miscarriages, and cancers.

Organic varieties tend to be smaller but are richer in flavour and possess good concentration of vitamins, minerals, and antioxidants.

THE VEGETABLES LISTED ALPHABETICALLY

Alfalfa sprouts
Alugbati
Arracacha
Artichoke
Arugula
Asparagus
Bamboo shoots
Baobab
Barley grass
Beans
Beets
Bell pepper
Bitter gourd
Bok choy
Broccoli
Broccoli rabe
Brussels sprouts
Cabbage
Cactus leaf
Caigua
Cardoon
Carrot
Cassava
Cauliflower
Celeriac
Celery
Chayote
Chicory
Collard greens
Corn
Cucumber
Daikon
Dandelion greens

Eggplant
Endive
Fennel
Fiddlehead
Garlic
Good King Henry
Green beans
Green peas
Horseradish
Jerusalem artichoke
Jicama
Kai-lan
Kale
Kohlrabi
Komatsuna
Lamb's quarters
Leeks
Lettuce
Lotus root
Luffa
Mache
Malabar gourd
Malanga
Mallow
Mashua
Molokhia
Moringa
Mushroom
Mustard greens
Oca
Okra
Onion
Parsley

Parsnip
Parwal
Potato
Pumpkin
Purslane
Radicchio
Radish
Red orach
Rhubarb
Rutabaga
Samphire
Scallions
Sea beet
Sea vegetables
Shallots
Soybean
Spinach
Squash
Sweet potato
Sweet chard
Taro
Tinda
Tomato
Turnip
Ulluco
Wasabi
Water chestnut
Watercress
Water spinach
Wheatgrass
Yacon
Yam

ALFALFA SPROUTS

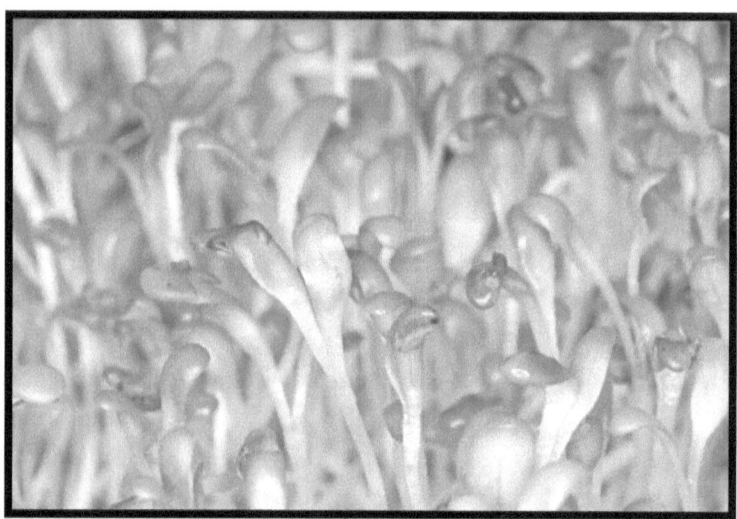

Alfalfa sprout is a member of the pea family, making it a legume. Alfalfa sprouts are derived from alfalfa seeds and are harvested before they become a full-grown plant. They have a mild flavour and are most often used in salads and sandwiches.

Alfalfa sprouts are the most nutrient-dense form of sprouts because their seeds produce long roots that reach deep into the earth to access trace elements and minerals. They are a rich source of fibre, protein, vitamins (K, A, C, E, B), minerals (calcium, magnesium, phosphorus, Iron, potassium, zinc), and antioxidants (beta-carotene, isoflavones, saponins, chlorophyll).

Some of the benefits of including alfalfa sprouts in our diets include the following:

- High fibre, high protein, no fat, and low calorie make it ideal to include it in our dieting programme.
- An amino acid, L-canavanine, present in alfalfa sprouts may fight against leukaemia and several other cancers such as pancreatic, colon, and breast cancers.

+ Antioxidants protect cells by fighting free radicals prohibiting cell oxidation, thus preventing chronic diseases.
+ Saponins stimulate immune system to fight infections by increasing the activity of natural killer cells.
+ Saponins lower production of inflammatory toxins in the gut.
+ Saponins lower blood cholesterol and blood pressure, thus preventing atherosclerosis, which could lead to heart attack or stroke.
+ Phytoestrogens present in alfalfa sprouts may increase bone formation and prevent osteoporosis.

ALUGBATI

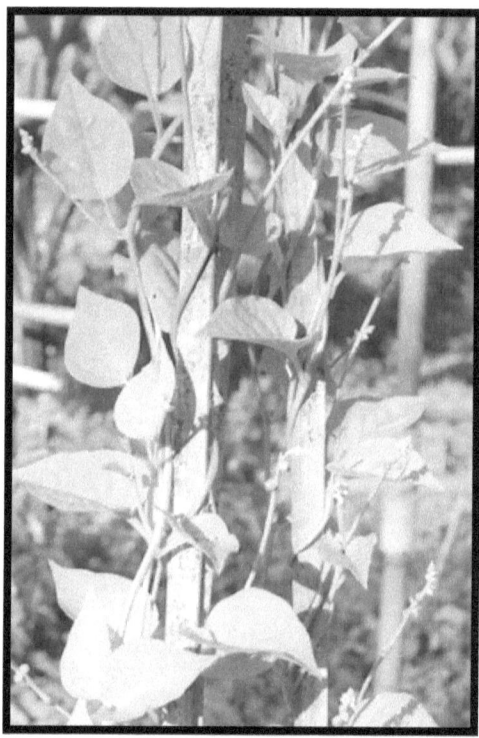

Alugbati is a common plant in the Philippines, where it is used as a vegetable and herbal medicine. It is used as a substitute for spinach and is also called Malabar spinach or Ceylon spinach although it is not spinach at all. The leaves and stems are used in salads, soups, stews, curries, stir-fries, and tofu diets or used as thickeners.

The leaves are heart-shaped, succulent, large, and grassy. The stem is red; hence, it is named red vine. The stem has a very mucilaginous texture. It bears green to dark red fruits.

Alugbati is a good source of fibre, vitamins A, B, and C, iron, calcium, and saponins. Saponins act as phytochemicals, which fight cancers and cardiovascular diseases. It is a diuretic and has a mild laxative effect. Alugbati is used to treat headache, inflammation, and ulcer.

Arracacha (White Carrot)

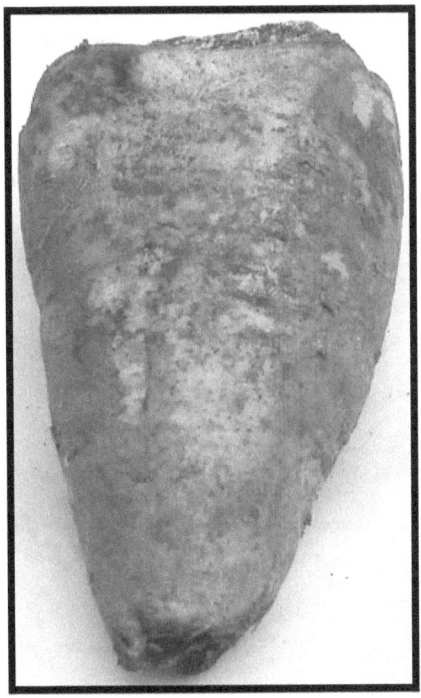

Arracacha is a starchy root vegetable, which originated in India. It is very popular in South America. It is very similar to carrot, hence nicknamed 'white carrot'. It is related to celery and carrot. The colour varies from white to yellow to purple. The taste is like a blend of celery, cabbage, and roasted chestnut. The leaves are dark green to purple and look like parsley.

Arracacha cannot be eaten raw but is used in soups, desserts, baby formulas, and used as thickeners. The boiled root is used as a boiled potato, but it has distinctive aroma and flavour. The young leaves can be used in salads or used as a cooking vegetable.

Arracacha is a rich source of fibre, vitamin C, and iron. The yellow variety is rich in carotenoids too. Because the starch granules in arracacha are very small, they are easily digested and thus are excellent for babies, elderly, and those suffering from indigestion.

ARTICHOKE

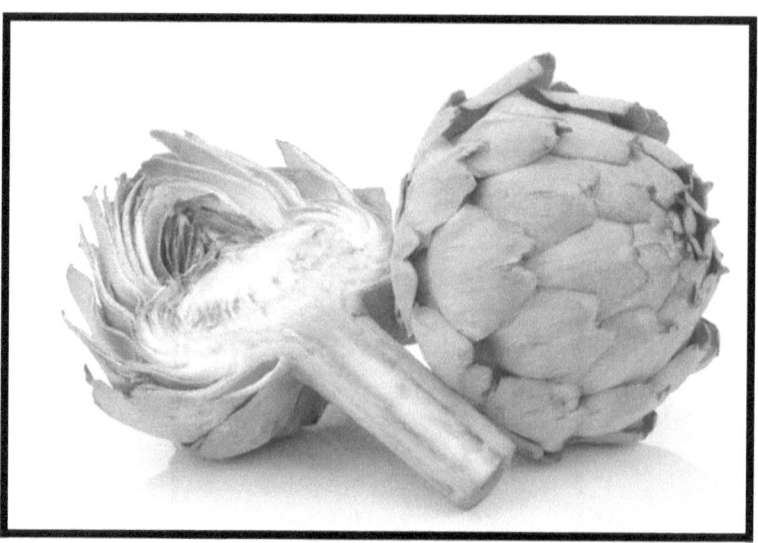

Artichoke was first developed in Sicily. Italy is now the largest producer of artichoke. Romans and Greeks used it as a vegetable in salads 2,000 years ago. The edible part of the plant is the flower base. It can be boiled, stir-fried, or added to pizza and pasta dishes. The word 'artichoke' was derived from *articicco*, which means fine cone.

Artichoke is a rich source of fibre, magnesium, potassium, folic acid, and powerful antioxidants (quercetin, rutin, anthocyanin, cynariniluteolin, silynarin). The antioxidant capacity of artichoke exceeds all other vegetables. The edible leaves of artichoke contain inulin, inulase, and cynarin.

Some of the benefits of eating artichoke include the following:

- It induces cell death and lowers cell proliferation in some cancers, such as leukemia and cancers of prostate, breast, and intestine.
- Cynarin increases bile flow, treats liver ailments, and improves liver function test.
- It improves digestion and relieves bloating and flatulence.

- It regulates blood glucose level, thus useful in diabetics.
- It lowers the pain of arthritis and gout.
- It is effective in the treatment of asthma.
- It has diuretic effect and rids the body of excessive fluids.
- It cures constipation by its high fibre content and increasing bile flow.
- It lowers blood pressure by its high potassium content.
- It prevents atherosclerosis by lowering bad cholesterol (LDL) and increasing good cholesterol (HDL).
- It aids in the treatment of irritable bowel syndrome.
- It increases libido and sex drive.
- It is effective in the treatment of migraine headaches.
- Because of their positive effects on the liver, artichoke leaves treat hangover.
- Extracts of its leaves are useful in treating bad odour, pruritus, oedema, and hair fall.

ARUGULA (ROCKET)

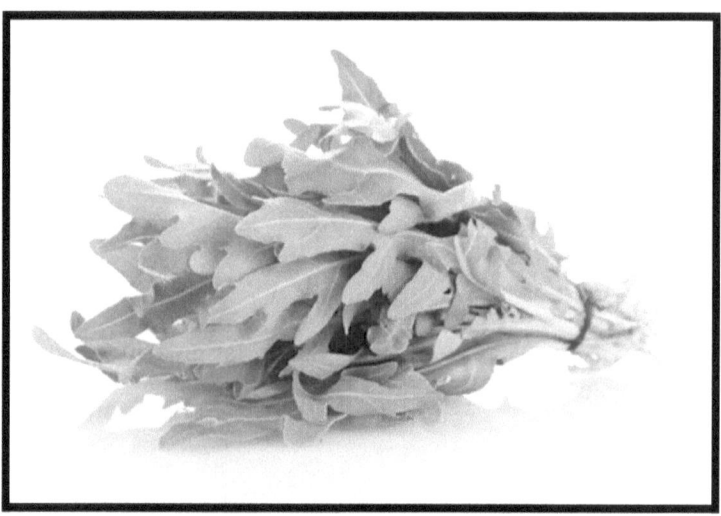

Arugula is a cruciferous, dark green vegetable belonging to the mustard family, like cauliflower, kale, and radish. It is native to the Mediterranean region. It has a rich peppery and pungent taste and is used in salads.

Arugula is a good source of fibre, vitamins (A, B, C, K), minerals (zinc, copper, iron, calcium, magnesium, phosphorus, potassium, manganese), carotenoids (beta-carotene, lutein, zeaxanthin), phytochemicals (indoles, thiocyanates, isothiocyanates, sulphoraphanes) and glucosinolates, which are converted in the body to isocyanates.

Health benefits of arugula exceed most of the greens, and it tastes great raw, unlike most of the cruciferous vegetables.

The phytochemicals in arugula counter carcinogenic effects of oestrogen and thus benefit against breast, cervical, ovarian, prostate, and colon cancers.

Isocyanates regulate immune function.

The phytochemicals contain lots of compounds, which enable the body's cells to detoxify by helping the liver create more of the antioxidant glutathione. High content of vitamins K and C, calcium, magnesium, manganese, and zinc contribute to positive bone build-up.

Iron, copper, and vitamin C in arugula aid in preventing anaemia.

High carotenoids in arugula prevent night blindness and macular degeneration.

Low oxalate content, as compared to other leafy greens such as spinach, is favourable to calcium absorption from the gut.

Asparagus
(Aristocrat of Vegetables)

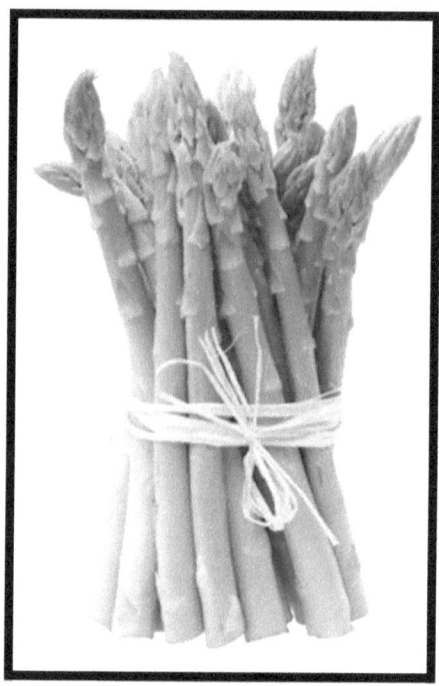

Asparagus belongs to the Lily family, of which more than 300 varieties exist, although only twenty of them are edible. Asparagus is native to Africa, Asia, and Europe and has been cultivated for thousands of years for its delicate texture and medicinal values. It has slender, succulent green or white or purple spears with a head. The finest texture and taste are in the tips. It can be eaten raw, steamed, stir-fried, pickled, or added to soups.

Asparagus is one of the most nutritionally balanced vegetable. It is rich in vitamins (B, A, C, E, K), minerals (calcium, magnesium, phosphorus, zinc, selenium, chromium, potassium, copper, manganese), protein, fibre, rutin (a compound that strengthens capillary walls), and amino acids (asparagines, glutathione, tryptophan).

Some of the health benefits of asparagus include the following:

- It has many antioxidants, such as vitamins (C, A, E), minerals (zinc, manganese, selenium) and glutathione.
- It has several anti-inflammatory compounds such as saponins, quercetin, and rutin.
- It contains inulin, which feeds the friendly bacteria that live in the large intestine.
- The high content of antioxidants, anti-inflammatory compounds, and chromium assist in glucose utilisation.
- It has the highest concentration of glutathione, which protects against many cancers such as colon, bladder, breast, prostate, lung, and ovarian cancers.
- Vitamin K, calcium, magnesium, phosphorus, and zinc aid in strong bone formation and prevention of osteoporosis.
- High folic acid, antioxidants, and anti-inflammatory compounds lower the risk of heart diseases.
- High vitamins A and C boost the immunity.
- B vitamins help in the metabolism of carbohydrates, fats, and proteins, boosting energy.
- It is an effective diuretic.
- Its high folic acid content prevents birth defects in the newborns.
- Its diuretic effect lowers water retention and bloating associated with menstruation.
- Its folic acid, iron, copper, and vitamin C help in preventing anaemia.
- It aids in increasing flow of milk in the nursing mothers.
- It has the essential nutrients which aid in growing healthy hair.
- Tryptophan aids in relieving depression and insomnia.
- Vitamins A and B, protein, and glutathione are anti-ageing agents.

Amino acids and minerals in asparagus may ease hangovers and protect the liver cells from alcohol.

Asparagus has psychological effect on libido. Due to the shape of this vegetable, French call it asperge, meaning penis in slang.

Bamboo Shoots
(The King of Forest Vegetables)

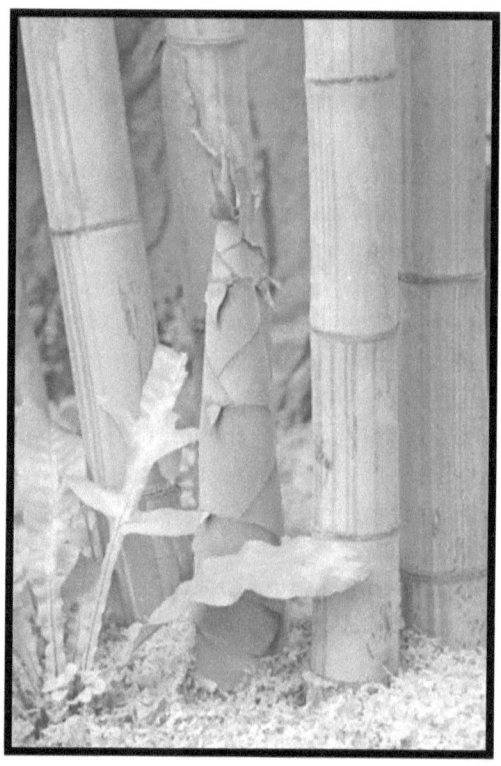

Bamboo shoot is a traditional Chinese forest vegetable, which has been in use for over 2,500 years. It is the sprout that springs out beside the plant. It is the largest, tallest, and fastest growing plant in the grass family. There are two types, namely, winter and spring shoots. The spring variety is larger and tougher than the winter variety. Bamboo shoots form an essential ingredient in dishes of many Asian countries. Bamboo shoots must be boiled before they can be consumed. They are used in snacks, curries, soups, salads, pickles, and fried rice.

Bamboo shoots are rich in fibre, protein with eight essential amino acids, essential fatty acids, vitamins (A, E, B), minerals (potassium, phosphorus, calcium, magnesium, manganese, zinc, copper, iron, chromium, selenium), and phytochemicals.

Health benefits of bamboo shoots include the following:

+ They contain phytosterols, similar to cholesterol, which inhibit absorption of cholesterol in the intestinal tract and thus help lower the LDL in the blood.
+ They improve digestion, increase appetite, and prevent constipation.
+ High potassium content lowers blood pressure.
+ The vital nutrients in bamboo shoot protect the body from several types of cancer.
+ Phytonutrients lower the risk of many chronic inflammatory diseases like arthritis and asthma.
+ Due to high antioxidant activity and the presence of phenolic compounds, bamboo shoots have antibiotic activity. They are used to clean wounds and sores.
+ They lower gallbladder spasms, which cause severe pain.
+ They speed up menstruation and labour in the last month of pregnancy.

Baobab (Kuka)

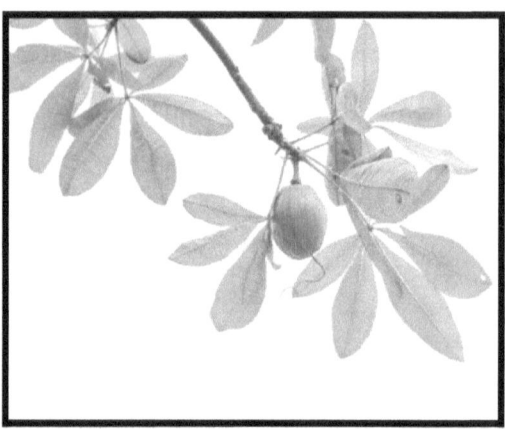

Boabab leaves are of African origin and are staple ingredients in African cuisine. It is commonly used in kuka soup and is used as a leaf vegetable like spinach. Kuka powder is mixed in salads and soups as a thickener.

Baobab is rich in potassium, calcium, vitamin C, carotenes, rhamnose, mucilage, tannins, catechins, and glutamic acid

Antioxidant

Anti-inflammatory

Anti-asthmatic

Anti-allergic

Antipyretic

Anti-perspiration

Mucolytic (expectorant for cough)

The powdered leaf is used to treat sores.

BARLEY GRASS

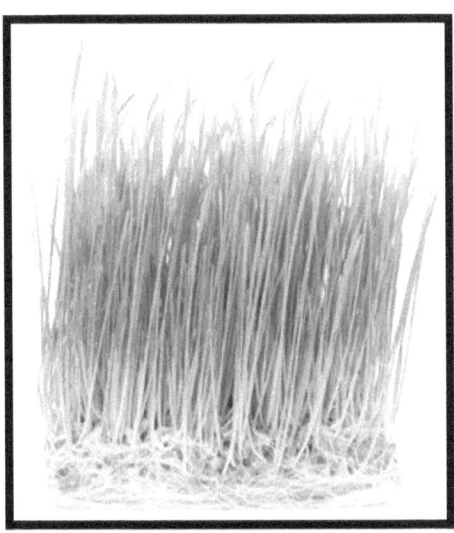

Barley grass is the young leaf of the barley plant harvested before it forms grain. Barley grass is more nutrient-dense than green leafy vegetables. Before consumption, barley grass is converted to juice or powder. The juice is more nutritious because heating denatures the healthy enzymes.

There is not much difference between the nutritional content of barley grass and wheat grass. They are both considered super foods because of their dense nutritional properties. Barley grass is rich in vitamins (A, C, B), minerals (potassium, calcium, magnesium, phosphorus, iron, copper, and manganese), amino acids, protein, enzymes, and chlorophyll.

Barley leaf extract has antioxidant activity due to its ability to scavenge free radicals.

It contains beta-sitosterol, which inhibits absorption of cholesterol from intestine and accelerates its catabolism to bile acid.

It is antibacterial.

It boosts immunity.

Chlorophyll, having similar structure to haemoglobin, has a role in blood formation.

It controls blood glucose level.

It neutralises toxins in the body.

It improves digestion.

The green barley leaves are strongly alkaline and neutralise the harmful effect of acidity of processed foods.

BEANS

Bean or pulse is a legume that belongs to the vegetable category of foods. There are about 14,000 species of beans available. Beans are one of the oldest cultivated crops dating back to over 7,000 years.

Beans are rich sources of B vitamins, fibre, protein, complex carbohydrates, phytochemicals, and minerals (iron, calcium, magnesium, phosphorus, manganese, copper, zinc, potassium). One cup of cooked bean provides twelve grams of fibre, equivalent to half of our daily requirement. Bean protein can be used as a substitute for meat if combined with other plant proteins, such as rice or bread, to make a complete protein, containing all the essential amino acids. Beans are low in calories and saturated fats and are devoid of cholesterol but are rich in flavonoid antioxidants. Darker-coloured beans have higher level of anthocyanins and, thus, higher antioxidant activity. The higher antioxidant activities are found in black beans, followed by red, brown, yellow, and white in that order. Red kidney beans have more antioxidant activity than even blueberries. Antioxidants fight off the free radicals and prevent diseases such as Alzheimer's, heart diseases, stroke, and some cancers, and they give beans anti-ageing properties.

There are many types of beans classified according to their colour, shape, and size. The nutritional values of most beans are quite similar, with the exception of anthocyanin level, as mentioned above.

Adzuki Beans (Azuki Beans)

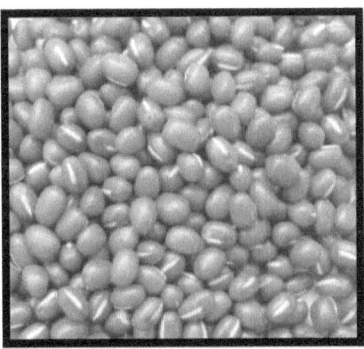

They are small, oval, reddish-brown beans with a thin white stripe down the side. It is native to China. It is somewhat sweet and has a delicate texture.

Anasazi Beans

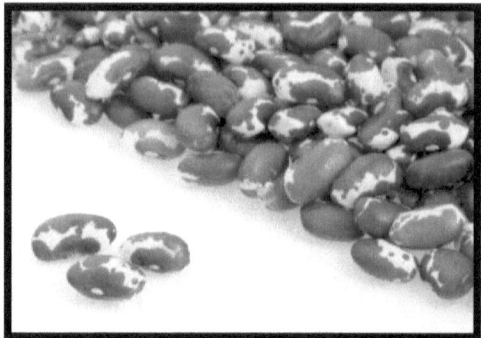

They are small, kidney-shaped, reddish-brown beans with white markings. It originated in New Mexico and is also called cave bean. They have mild sweet flavour and meaty texture.

Black Beans (Turtle Beans)

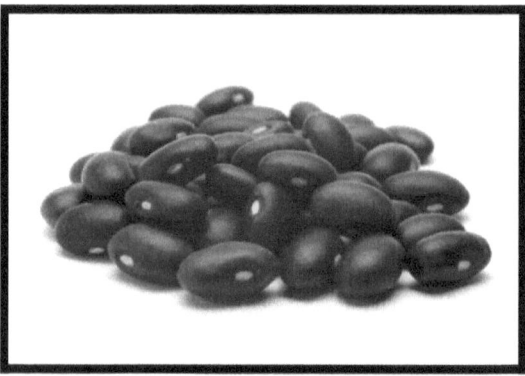

They are small, oval beans with earthy, sweet flavour and soft texture. They are popular in Latin American cuisine.

Black-Eyed Peas

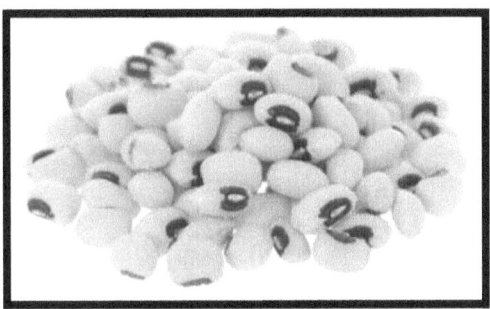

They are pea-sized, oval, ivory-coloured beans with a black 'eye'. They have mild, sweet, earthy taste, similar to mushrooms. They originated in East Asia.

Cannellini Beans (White Kidney Beans)

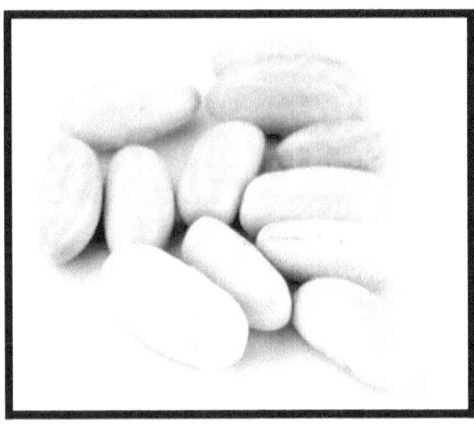

They are large white beans with firm texture and skin and a nutty flavour. They are very popular in Italy.

Chickpeas (Garbanzo Beans)

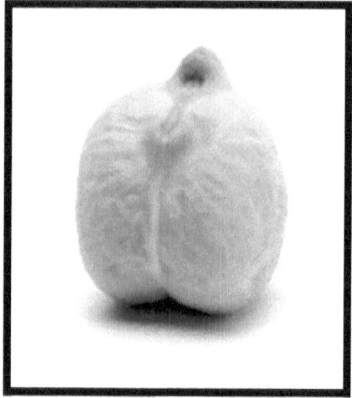

Chickpeas are large, round, cream—or green-coloured beans with nutty flavour and crunchy texture. It is an ancient bean, used for thousands of years in the Middle East (as hummus and falafel), India, Spain, Italy, and Latin America.

Corona Beans

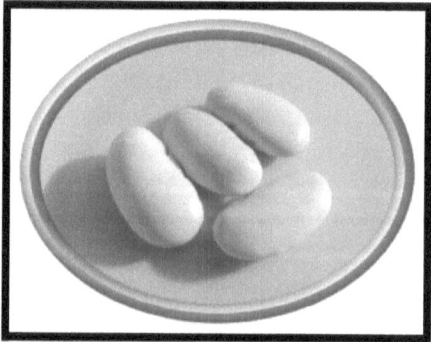

They are large, plump, and ivory-coloured beans with a rich flavour and a tender meaty texture. It is common in Italian cuisine.

Cranberry Beans (Borlotti Beans)

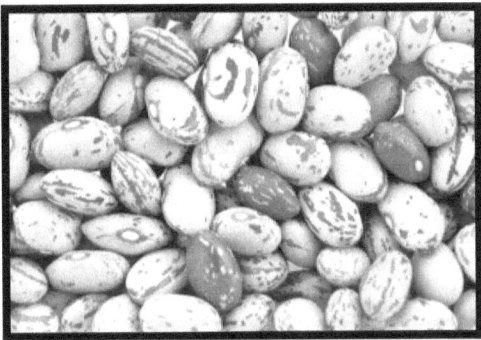

They are white beans with deep-red specks and have mild, nutty flavour similar to chestnuts.

Fava Beans (Broad Beans)

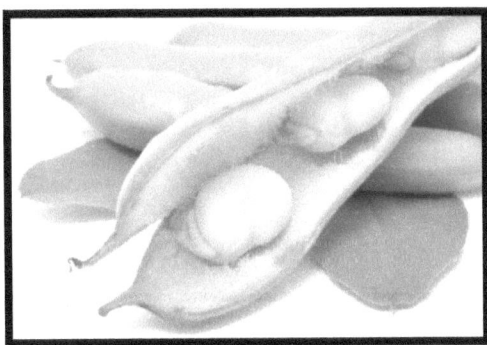

They are a member of the pea family. They are large, flattened, light-green, thick indigestible pods. They have delicious, meaty flavour and creamy texture. They are native to North Africa and South-West Asia and are very popular in Middle Eastern cuisine.

Flageolet Beans (Caviar of Beans)

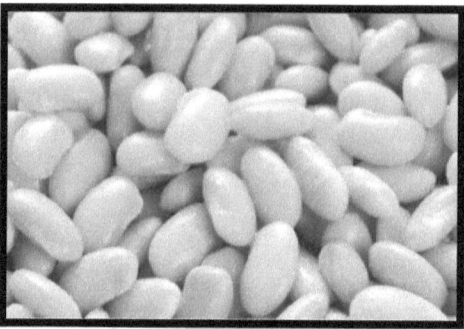

They are small, immature, kidney beans that have pale green colour, tender skin, and fine delicate flavour that grow in France.

Great Northern Beans

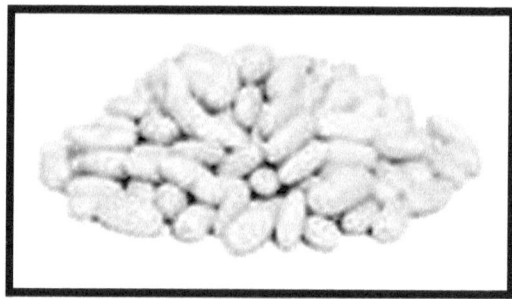

They are flat, kidney-shaped, medium-sized white beans with thin skin, delicate flavour and tender creamy flesh that grow in North America.

Haricot Beans (Navy Beans)

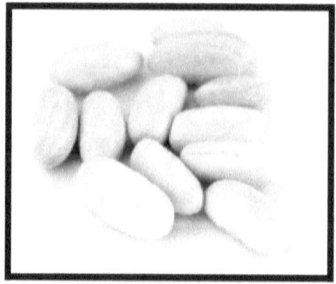

They are small, plump, and creamy-white with a mild flavour and smooth, buttery texture. They are widely used in Europe and South America.

Kidney Beans

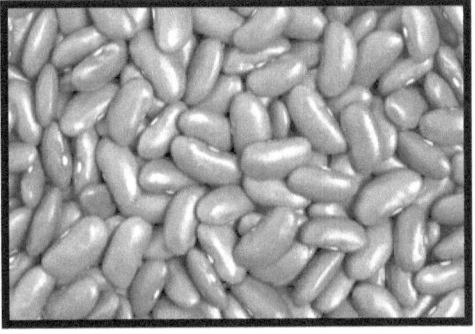

They are reddish-brown, kidney-shaped with a soft, creamy flesh.

Lentils

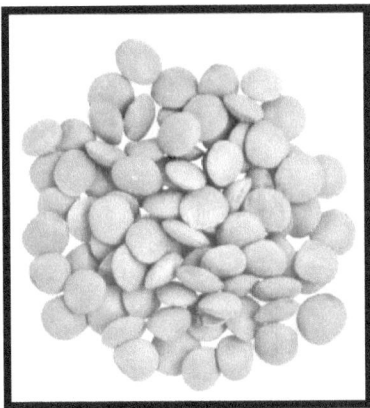

They are small, lens-shaped, flavourful legumes with a fine texture, ranging in colour from yellow to orange-red, green, brown, and black.

Lima Beans (Butter Beans)

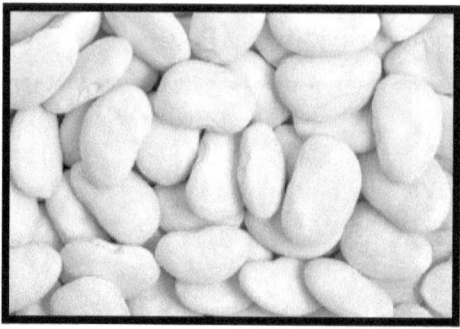

They are flat, oval, creamy-white with buttery, grainy, mushy texture and potato-like taste. Lima bean is named after Lima, Peru, where it was first cultivated.

Lupini Beans

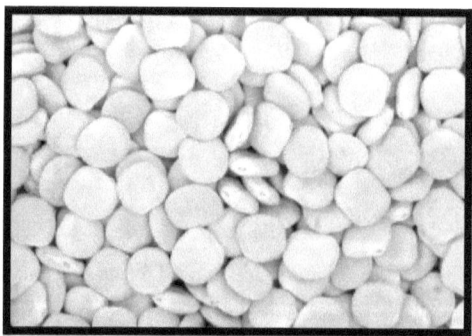

They are large, flat, round, yellow with a thick, tough skin, native to Italy.

Marrow Beans

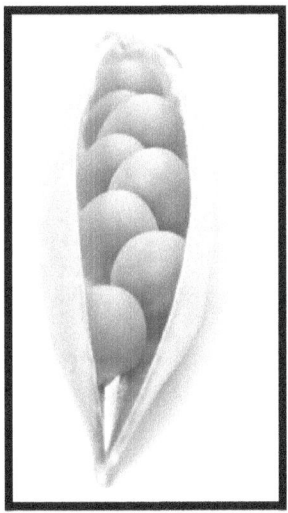

They are large, plump, white beans with a creamy texture and a flavour similar to smoked meat. They are of the Middle Eastern origin and are popular in Italy.

Mung Beans

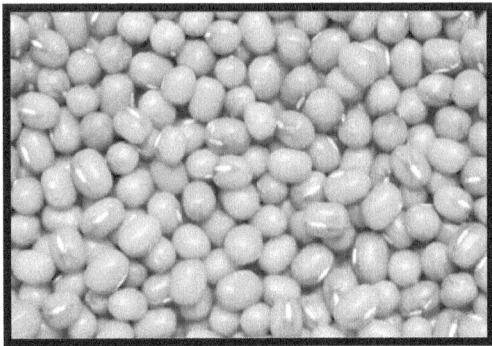

They are tiny, beautiful, golden-green beans, native to India.

Orca Beans

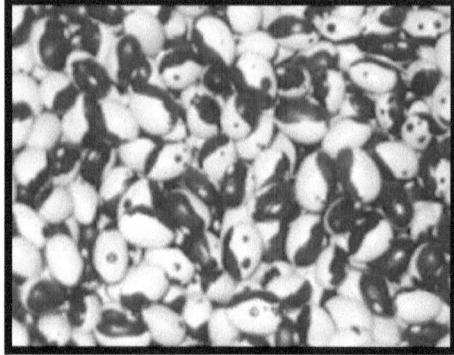

One half of the bean is pure white; the other half is shiny black. It is named after black and white killer whale, orca whale, and is native to Mexico.

Pink Beans (Chilli Beans)

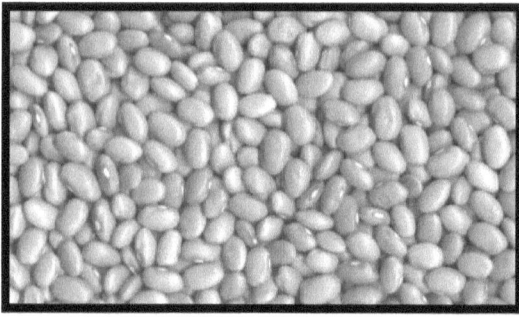

They are small, oval, pale-pink beans with a smooth, meaty texture and a mild sweet taste.

They are popular in Western America and the Caribbean.

Pinto Beans

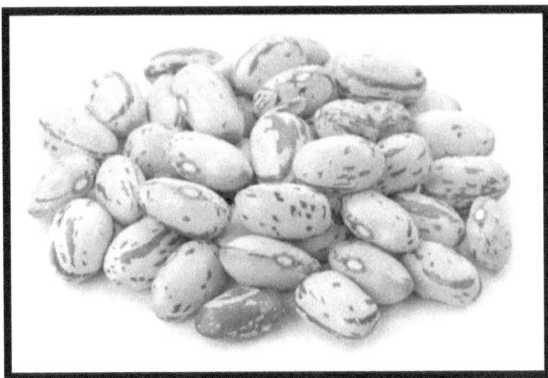

They are medium-sized, oval, beige with reddish-brown specks all over. Pinto is the Spanish word for 'painted'. It is grown in Latin America and south-west America.

Red Beans

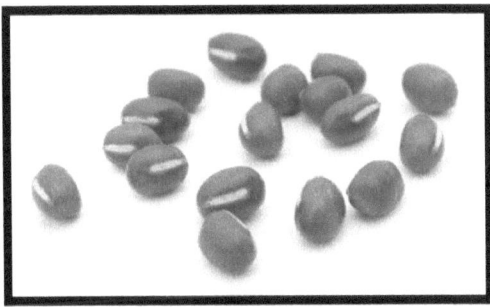

They are small, dark-red, and slightly sweet beans. They are smaller and rounder than red kidney beans.

Shelly Beans

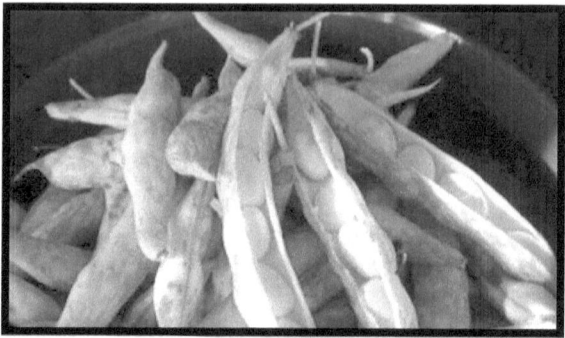

They are the mature green beans that grow inside the green bean pod.

Split Peas

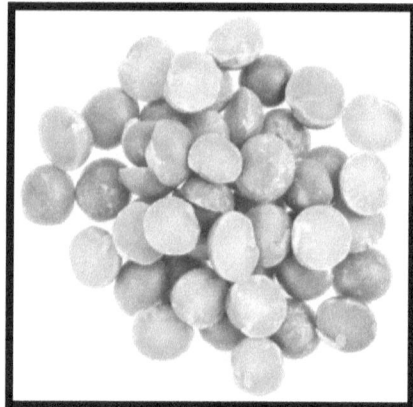

They are small, green or yellow halved peas that have earthy flavour and creamy texture.

BEETS

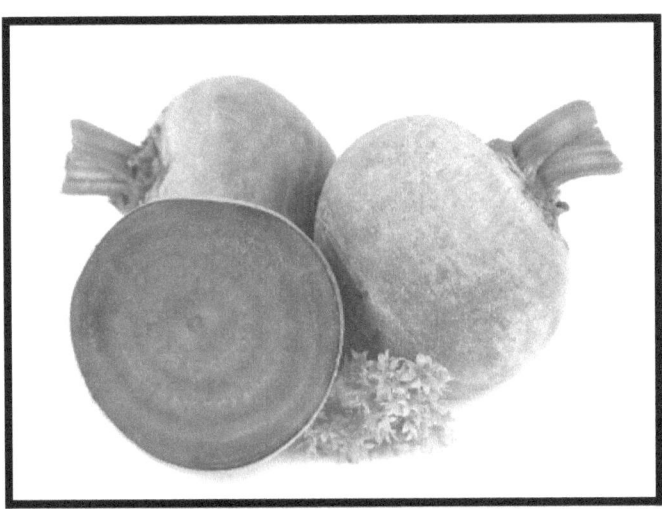

Beets originated in prehistoric times in North Africa, and they were domesticated in the Mediterranean regions. There are three varieties of table beets: red, which contains betacyanin, yellow, which contains betaxanthin, and white speckled with pink. Sugar beets are larger with higher sugar content than table beets (80% versus 20%).

Beetroots can be cooked, pickled, roasted, sautéed, juiced, used in salad, or made into wine.

Beets are rich sources of folic acid, fibre, potassium, magnesium, manganese, copper, iron, phosphorus, and tryptophan. Beet leaves or greens are rich in vitamins A and C, lutein, and zeaxanthin.

Some of the benefits of eating beet include the following:

Betaine lowers homocysteine level in the blood, which could be harmful to blood vessels.

The phytochemicals lower the risk of several kinds of cancers, including colon, stomach, lung, breast, prostate, and testicular cancers.

High sugar content provides great amount of quick energy.

The high nitrates in beets are converted in the body to nitrous oxide, which acts as a vasodilator, increasing blood flow to genital areas. Thus, it has an effect similar to Viagra. Ancient Romans used beets for their aphrodisiac effect. Moreover, boron in beets increases the production of human sex hormones.

Iron and copper in beets aid in preventing anaemia.

Betaine stimulates liver function.

The high fibre content prevents constipation and piles.

High folic acid content aids in DNA synthesis and prevents neural tube defect in newborns.

High tryptophan content gives relief from depression and insomnia.

It has a powerful anti-ageing effect.

BELL PEPPER (SWEET PEPPER)

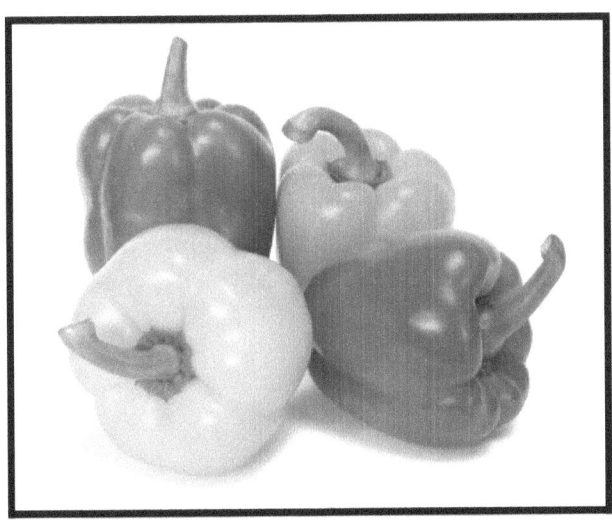

Bell pepper is native to Mexico. Both chilli pepper and sweet pepper belong to the capsicum family. Because bell pepper is not 'hot', it is not considered as a spice. Bell pepper is regarded as a vegetable but is actually botanically a 'fruit'. It has sweet, crunchy taste and a thick, waxy, fleshy texture, enclosing numerous tiny, white, circular seeds that cling to a central core. The reason behind its sweetness is having only a small amount of capsaicin. Bell pepper can be found in a variety of colours that vary in flavours. All the varieties start as green, but as they mature, their colours turn to yellow, orange, red, black, and purple and become sweeter and more nutritious.

Bell pepper is rich in fibre, vitamins (A, C, K, B6, and folic acid), minerals (potassium, magnesium, manganese, and molybdenum), lutein, cumaric acid, chlorogenic acid, zeaxanthin, cryptoxanthin, and lycopene in red variety.

Some of the benefits of eating bell pepper include the following:

+ It lowers the risk of several types of cancer, including gastric, oesophageal, prostatic, ovarian, breast, cervix, bladder, pancreatic, and lung cancers.

- It has anti-inflammatory effects and lowers the severity of arthritis and asthma.
- Vitamins B6 and folic acid lower the level of blood homocysteine that could damage the blood vessels. Vitamin C, flavonoids, and capsaicin lower the risk of heart attack and stroke. High fibre content lowers blood cholesterol level.
- Capsaicin lowers the risk of stomach ulcer by killing the bacteria that causes ulcer.
- Lutein, zeaxanthin, vitamin A, and vitamin C slow down the development of cataract and macular degeneration.
- High antioxidant content boosts immunity.
- High vitamin B6 and folic acid make bell pepper an ideal vegetable during pregnancy.

Bitter Gourd (Bitter Melon)

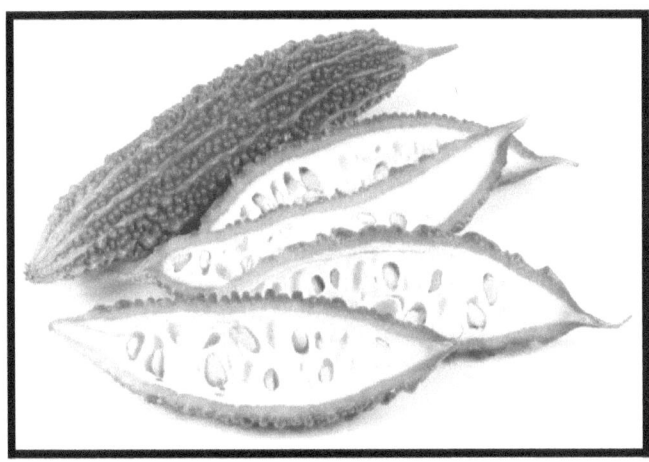

Bitter gourd originated in India, but now, it is a very popular vegetable throughout Asia. It is a member of the same family as squash and cucumber. It looks like a cucumber with ugly bumps all over it. It is among the most bitter of all vegetables, hence the name bitter gourd. It comes in a variety of shapes and sizes. The shape could be oval or oblong with a pointed tip. The colour varies from light to dark green. The flesh is white when immature but turns red at maturity. It is usually consumed cooked or is used in soups.

Bitter gourd is rich in fibre, vitamins (C, B3, B5, B6, and B9), minerals (iron, zinc, potassium, manganese, and magnesium), flavonoids (carotenes, lutein, and zeaxanthin), and phytochemicals (charantin and polypeptide-p).

Some of the health benefits of bitter gourd include the following:

+ Charantin and polypeptide-p act as insulin, lowering blood glucose level in type 2 diabetes.
+ High carotenoid content aids in healthy vision.
+ It stimulates digestive system and prevents constipation and piles.

- It lowers the risk of breast cancer.
- It boosts immunity.
- It acts as a blood purifier.
- It is effective in the treatment of psoriasis.
- It is an effective remedy for hangover.
- It prevents neural tube defect in offspring.
- It is used in the treatment of gastric ulcer and colitis.

Bok Choy

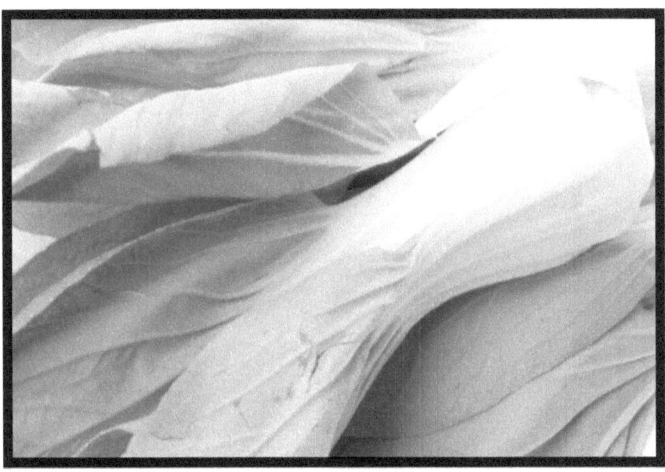

Bok Choy is called Chinese cabbage, but it actually is chard. It is a member of the brassica family and is related to turnip. It is made up of dark-green leaves similar to spinach with firm, bright, white stalks. It is crunchy and has mild taste. It can be eaten as stew, soup, salad, or stir-fried.

Bok Choy is a rich source of fibre, vitamins (A, C, K, B, and D), minerals (calcium, potassium, manganese, iron, and magnesium), and indoles.

It lowers the risk of breast, colon, prostate, and lung cancers.

It boosts immunity.

It prevents Alzheimer's disease.

It is a bone builder.

It prevents anaemia.

It aids in vision health.

It lowers the risk of type 2 diabetes.

It prevents constipation.

It is beneficial for heart health.

BROCCOLI

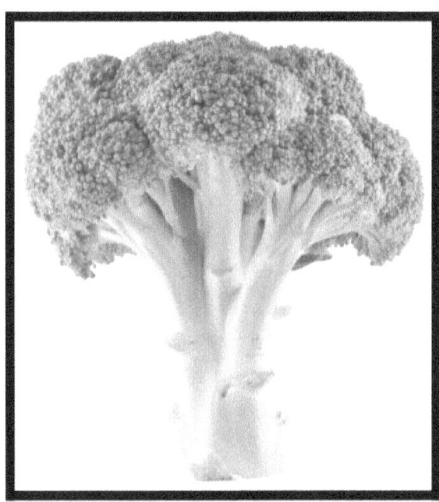

Broccoli is a cruciferous vegetable that belongs to the cabbage family. The large, green flower head of broccoli is used as a vegetable, and the thick stalk is edible too. It resembles cauliflower. Broccoli dates back to ancient Rome. The name 'broccoli' was derived from the Italian word *brachium*, which means branch. Broccoli can be eaten raw or cooked.

Broccoli is rich in fibre, protein, tryptophan, omega-3 fatty acids, phytochemicals (isothiocyanates, glucoraphanin), vitamins (C, A, K, B), and minerals (phosphorus, manganese, zinc, iron, potassium).

Glucoraphanin is converted in the body to sulphoraphane that kills the bacteria responsible for gastric ulcer, the precursor of stomach cancer.

Indoles found in broccoli prevent breast, cervical, and prostate cancers.

Vitamin B6, folic acid, carotenoids, omega-3 fatty acids, and fibre lower the risk of heart diseases and stroke.

It aids in eye health.

It builds strong bones and prevents osteoporosis.

It has a flavonoid compound called kaempferol, which reduces allergic reactions.

Isothiocyanates and glucoraphanin control detoxification processes in the body.

It strengthens the immunity defence system.

BROCCOLI RABE (RAPINI, BROCCOLETTI)

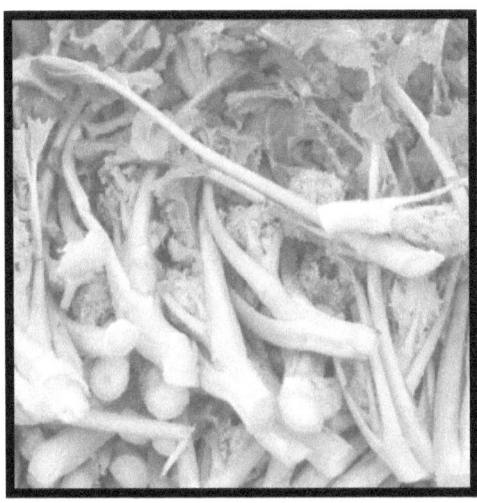

Rapini belongs to the cabbage family. It originated in the Mediterranean region and China as a descendent from a wild herb. It is the most popular vegetable in Hong Kong and is used very commonly in Italy. Rapini is an emerald-green, crispy, leafy vegetable with curly leaves and baby florets, which resemble broccoli, but it is more closely related to mustard greens and turnip greens. The taste is nutty, pungent and slightly bitter. The florets can be eaten along with the leaves.

Rapini is rich in vitamins (A, C, K, and folic acid), minerals (potassium, calcium, iron), fibre, and phytochemicals (sulphoraphane and indoles).

Sulpharophane and indoles defend against certain cancers, such as stomach, lung, colon, breast, and prostate cancers.

It protects against heart diseases and stroke.

It helps in bone formation.

Rapini contains sulphur in a compound called MSM, which assists in liver detoxification.

MSM also lowers the inflammation in arthritis.

It boosts immunity and fights infections.

Brussels Sprouts

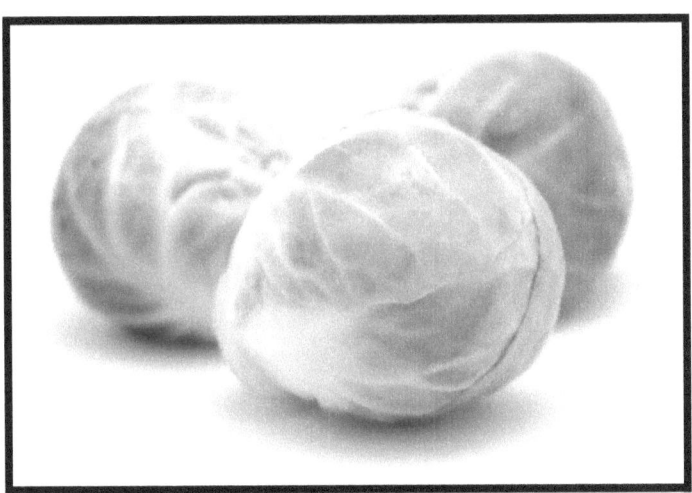

Brussels sprouts are a member of the cabbage family. It is actually not sprouts but small, leafy, green buds that resemble a miniature cabbage. It was probably first cultivated in Brussels, Belgium, from where it got its name.

Brussels sprouts are a very rich source of fibre, protein, omega-3 fatty acids, vitamins (C, A, K, folic acid), minerals (potassium, calcium, magnesium, phosphorus), and phytochemicals (indoles, sulphoraphane, isothioyanates, sinirain, lutein, zeaxanthin).

Phytochemicals lower the risk of several cancers, such as colon, breast, lung, prostate, ovarian, and endometrial cancers.

Vitamins A and C and omega-3 fatty acids help in getting healthy skin.

It aids in healthy vision.

It promotes bone health.

It prevents Alzheimer's disease.

Phytonutrients aid in preventing DNA damage.

It is a great aid in weight management programme.

Antioxidants and anti-inflammatory compounds lower the risk of heart diseases and stroke.

It boosts immunity and fights infection.

CABBAGE

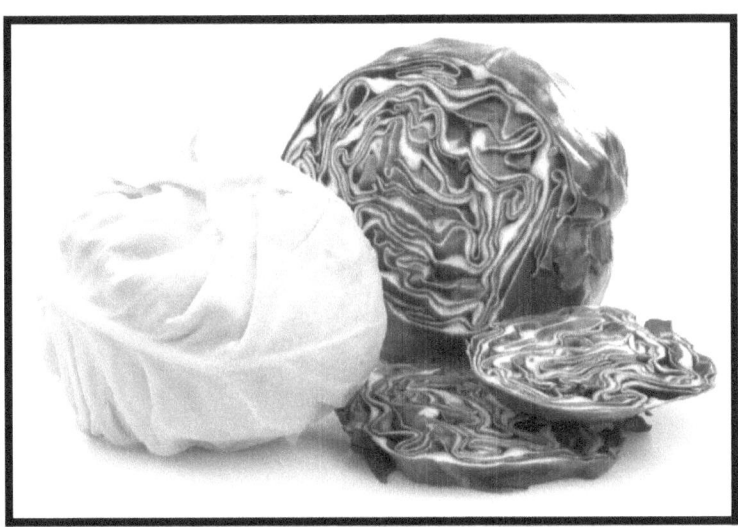

Cabbage belongs to the brassica family. The name 'cabbage' was derived from the French word *caboche*, meaning 'head'. Cabbage was domesticated in Europe over 2,000 years ago. There are more than 400 varieties of cabbage, varying in shape (round, conical), size (up to 3.5 Kg), and colour (white, green, purple, red).

Cabbage has stiff leaves superimposed one over another in compact layers, giving it a globular shape. The leaves can be flat or curly and tight or loose.

Savoy cabbage is a variety that originated in Italy and is the most tender and sweet of all the varieties. It has loose-wrinkled leaves.

Cabbage is a rich source of fibre, vitamins (C, K, B-complex, beta-carotene), minerals (calcium, magnesium, manganese, potassium), and phytochemicals (indoles, sulphoraphane, isothicyanates). Red and purple varieties contain anthocyanins, in addition to those mentioned above.

Phytonutrients lower the risk of breast, lung, stomach, and colon cancers.

It treats peptic ulcer.

It has cardioprotective effect.

It is useful in weight reduction programmes.

It helps in building strong bones and preventing osteoporosis.

High vitamin K prevents damage to the nerve cells, which could lead to Alzheimer's disease.

CACTUS LEAF (NOPALES)

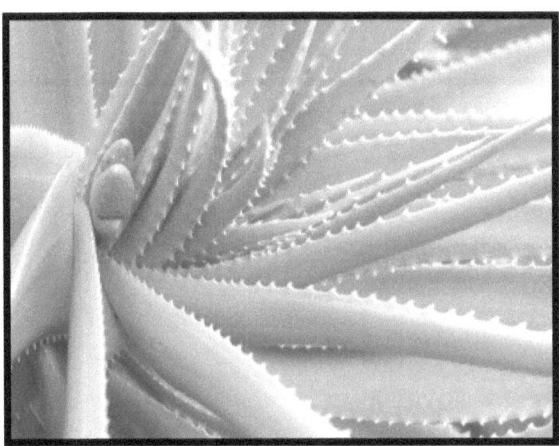

Cactus leaf is native to Mexico and has been a staple food in Latin America for centuries. The edible cactus has fleshy, oval, green or purple leaves (pads or paddles), with a soft, crunchy texture, which becomes sticky, like okra, after cooking. It tastes similar to asparagus, green beans, or green pepper. It is a common vegetable served in salads, and it is boiled, sautéed, steamed, or stir-fried.

Cactus leaf is a rich source of fibre, vitamins (A, C, folic acid), minerals (calcium, iron, magnesium, potassium, phosphorus), and flavonoid antioxidants.

Cactus leaves are low in calories (only four calories per serving) and thus are useful in dieting programmes.

The high fibre content lowers cholesterol, blood pressure, and blood glucose level.

Flavonoids lower the risk of colon, liver, breast, and prostate cancers.

Caigua
(Wild Cucumber, Lady's Slipper)

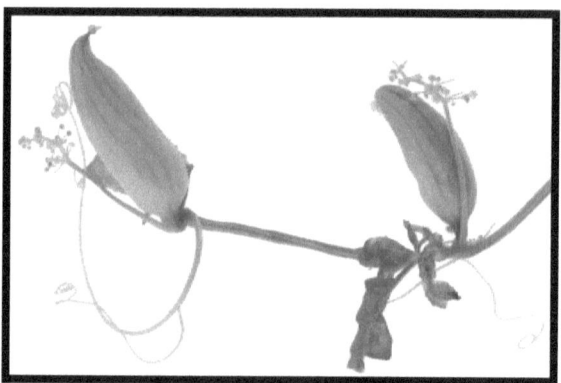

Caigua is a slender, tropical vine native to Peru, which produces pale to dark green, long, irregular, flat, soft, hollow fruit with a curved tip. It resembles cucumber but is hollow inside, like bell pepper, with several black seeds attached to a placenta. It can be eaten raw in salads, pickled, or stuffed, hence the name 'stuffing cucumber'.

Caigua is rich in fibre, vitamins (C, B1, B2), minerals (calcium, magnesium, iron, manganese, and potassium), sterols, and luteolin.

Sitosterol in caigua lowers LDL and increases HDL and, thus, cleans arteries and lowers blood pressure.

Luteolin controls blood glucose level.

It is a diuretic.

It has high anti-inflammatory properties and relieves arthritic pain.

It aids in digestion.

It can be used in weight reduction management.

CARDOON
(CARDONI, ARTICHOKE THISTLE)

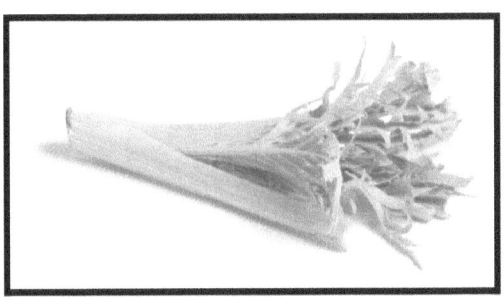

Cardoon is the tall member of the thistle family, related to artichoke, and looks like giant celery. It resembles thick, wide, spiny greenish-grey celery stalks with prickly silver-blue leaves. Cardoon is of the Mediterranean origin and has been cultivated in Europe since fifteenth century.

Cardoon has a subtle sweet taste of artichokes and celery with a hint of bitterness, which disappears after cooking. Cardoon can be eaten raw, braised, fried, baked, or made into soups.

Cardoon is a rich source of fibre, vitamin C, iron, calcium, potassium, magnesium, copper, manganese, phosphorus, flavonoids (apigenin, luteolin), and antioxidants (sillymarin, caffeic acid, ferulic acid).

Cardoon is a very low-caloric vegetable, which is ideal for losing weight.

Cynarin and sesquiterpene, which impart bitterness to cardoon, lower blood cholesterol level by inhibiting its synthesis and by increasing its excretion in the bile.

The antioxidants in cardoon protect cellular particles from oxidative damage caused by free radicals.

Apigenin lowers the risk of ovarian cancer and leukaemia and helps in relieving gout by preventing the build-up of uric acid.

CARROT

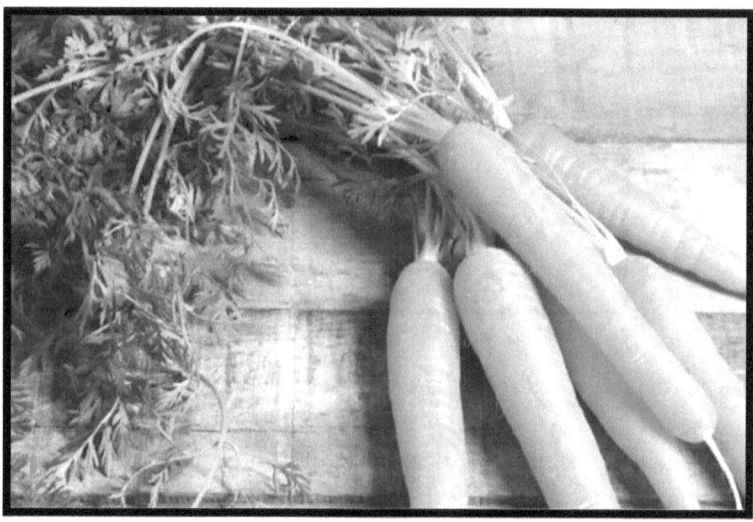

Carrot is a horn-like root vegetable, which originated in Iran and Afghanistan. It has been bred to decrease its bitterness and the fibrous core. Although carrot is usually orange in colour, it can come in other varieties, namely, purple, red, yellow, or white. It has a crisp, sweet taste and can be eaten raw, boiled, fried, juiced, or added to soups, stews, or desserts. Carrot is the second most popular vegetable after potato.

Carrot is a very rich source of fibre, alpha and beta-carotenes, vitamins (A, C, K, and B), potassium, and phytochemicals.

The presence of falcarinol and falcarindiol decrease the risk of lung, breast, and colon cancers.

Carotenoids prevent night blindness, senile cataract, and macular degeneration.

It lowers cholesterol and prevents heart diseases and stroke.

Antioxidant effects of carotenes help slow down the ageing of cells, thus preventing premature wrinkling and skin pigmentation, and improve skin tone.

The high vitamin A helps the liver in flushing out the toxins from the body.

The high vitamin K functions in blood clot formation, bone build-up, and the prevention of Alzheimer's disease.

The high vitamin C improves immune system, aids in iron absorption, combats free radical, and aids in the formation of strong bones and teeth.

The high vitamin B-complex acts as cofactors in metabolism.

The high potassium lowers blood pressure and stroke, improves the health of heart muscle and nervous system, and regulates electrolyte absorption from the gut.

The high fibre (two grams per carrot) promotes bowel movement, regulates weight management, and controls blood glucose.

CASSAVA (TAPIOCA, YUCCA)

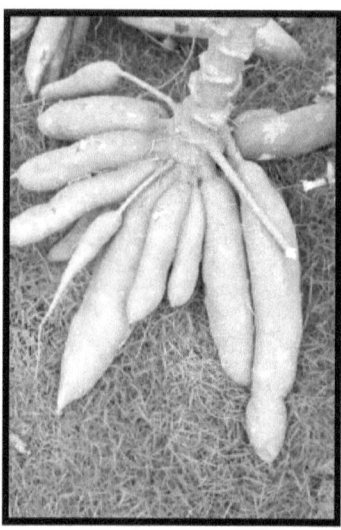

Cassava is a long, tubular root with a thin, brown skin and white flesh. Cassava is native to South America and is the staple crop in Africa, Asia, and South America. Cassava is the third largest source of food calories in the tropics after rice and corn.

Cassava can grow in poor soil and can withstand severe drought. The weight of cassava root can vary from one to several pounds. Cassava has two varieties: sweet and bitter.

Cassava is rich in carbohydrates, mainly starch, which is the major source of energy. With the exception of sugar cane and sugar beet, cassava is the highest source of carbohydrates. Cassava also contains fibre, vitamin C, calcium, and phosphorus, but it is a poor source of protein. Thus, those who depend solely on cassava could risk development of protein deficiency, called kwashiorkor.

Cassava contains cyanogenic glycosides, which can be broken down to release the toxin hydrogen cyanide. Hence, cassava must be properly prepared before consumption.

Cauliflower (Cabbage Flower)

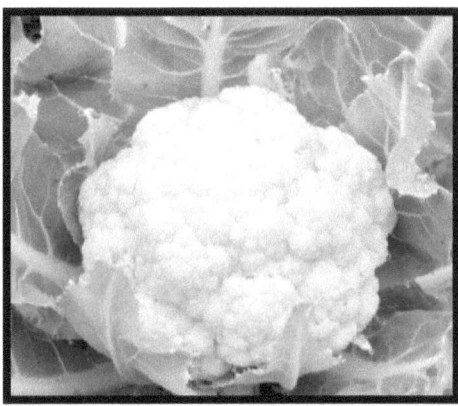

Cauliflower is one of the several cruciferous vegetables. It is the descendent of wild cabbage that originated in the Mediterranean region. The name 'cauliflower' comes from Latin caulis 'cabbage' and flower. The most available variety has white colour, but green, purple, and orange varieties are also available. Cauliflower is a member of the 'white' family of vegetables, which includes mushrooms, onion, and garlic. Like broccoli, cauliflower is made up of tightly clustered florets but stops at the bud stage. Cauliflower lacks chlorophyll, which gives broccoli its green colour; because the large leaves of cauliflower shield it from sunrays.

Cauliflower can be eaten raw, cooked, or stir-fried.

Cauliflower is a rich source of fibre, vitamins (C, K, and B), minerals (manganese, phosphorus, magnesium, and potassium), phytochemicals (indoles, sulphoraphane), protein, tryptophan, and omega-3 fatty acids.

White vegetables lower the risk of stroke more than the coloured vegetables.

The antioxidants vitamin C, manganese, carotenoids, and phytochemicals lower the risk of chronic diseases, such as heart diseases, stroke, and several forms of cancer like prostate, cervical, ovarian, and breast cancers.

The anti-inflammatory compounds vitamin K, omega-3 fatty acids, and phytochemicals lower the risk of inflammatory-mediated diseases, such as arthritis, asthma, and certain bowel diseases.

The presence of glucoraphin in cauliflower has a protective effect on stomach lining, preventing the bacterium H. pylori, which causes stomach ulcer and cancer.

Cauliflower contains detoxification enzymes.

Celeriac (Root Celery)

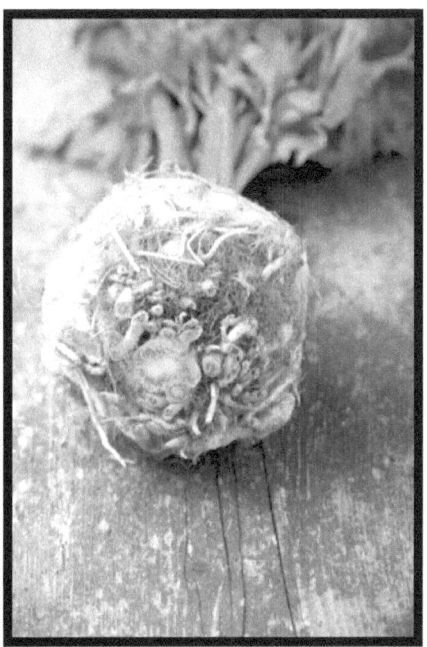

Celeriac is a winter root vegetable that originated in Northern Europe and the Mediterranean zone. It is a closely related variety of the common leaf celery, grown for its knobby underground root. Celeriac belongs to the carrot family. It has a coarse knobby outer surface with numerous small rootlets. It has a white smooth flesh that tastes like stalks of celery and has a nutty overtone.

Celeriac can be eaten raw or cooked, stewed, roasted, mashed, or added to soups.

Celeriac is a rich source of fibre, vitamins (K, C, and B6), and minerals (potassium, manganese, magnesium, iron, copper, calcium, zinc, selenium).

It has low caloric content and is free from fat and cholesterol.

Its high fibre content helps in proper digestion, prevention of constipation, and lowering of blood cholesterol.

It contains several polyacetylene antioxidants that have shown activity against colon cancer and acute lymphoblastic leukaemia (ALL).

Its high vitamin K increases bone mass by promoting osteotrophic activities in the bones and prevents Alzheimer's disease by limiting neuronal damage in the brain.

Phosphorus is required for cellular metabolism, buffer system, and bone health.

Iron and copper are involved in blood formation.

Its diuretic effect helps in eliminating excess fluids.

It is a good appetizer.

CELERY

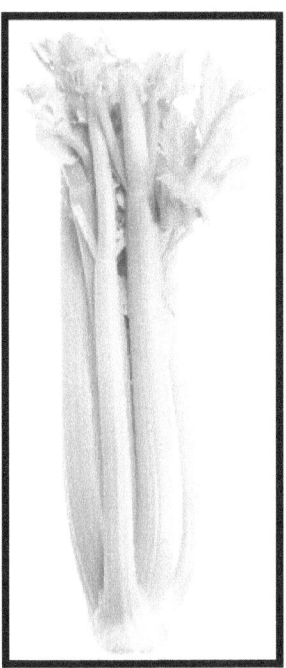

Celery is a crunchy, slightly salty vegetable that belongs to the umbelliferae family, which also includes celeriac, fennel, dill, carrot, parsley, and parsnip. Celery consists of stalks with leaf tips that are arranged in a conical shape joined at a common base.

Celery originated in the Mediterranean region.

Celery is considered a super vegetable because it has so many valuable nutrients and medicinal benefits. It is rich in fibres, vitamins (K, C, B, A), minerals (potassium, molybdenum, manganese, calcium, phosphorus, silicon, iron, magnesium), tryptophan, carotenoids (beta-carotene, lutein, zeaxanthin), phytosterols, flavonoids (apigenin, luteolin, quercetin), phthalides, coumarins, polyacetylenes, and phenolic acids.

Phenolic acids block the action of prostaglandins, which stimulate the growth of cancerous tumours. Phthalides and polyacetylenes detoxify carcinogens.

The antioxidant coumarins enhance the activity of certain white blood cells and, thus, support the immune system's ability to eliminate the harmful cells. High vitamin C also assists in boosting immunity.

Phthalides lower blood pressure by relaxing the muscle tissue in artery walls and increasing the blood flow. It lowers the stress hormones that can cause blood vessels to constrict.

Phytochemicals and fibre lower blood cholesterol level.

The presence of silicon, calcium, magnesium, phosphorus, manganese, and vitamin K help in building strong bones.

Celery has a diuretic effect and rids the body of excess fluids. It also removes uric acid crystals that build around joints, thus relieving swelling and pain.

Celery has anti-inflammatory effects and helps to lower the arthritic pain and asthma attacks.

Luteolin lowers the level of plaque-forming protein in the brain, thus preventing the onset of Alzheimer's disease.

The phytochemicals in celery have mild oestrogenic properties, which alleviate menopausal symptoms, such as hot flashes, heart disease, and osteoporosis.

The presence of coumarins tones the vascular system and relieves migraine. Phthalides that lower blood pressure also limit migraine attacks.

Tryptophan in celery is useful for insomniacs.

Celery has a very low caloric content (only nineteen calories per cup) and a high fibre, which will make it useful in weight reduction diets.

Celery seeds are found in flowers and have a strong, pleasant smell. They contain volatile oils (the cause of aroma), flavonoids (the cause of colours), coumarins (the cause of blood thinning), and linoleic acid (an omega-6 fatty acid). Celery seeds are used as diuretic and to treat cystitis and urethritis, to treat arthritis and gout, to lower blood pressure and cholesterol, to abort muscle spasms, and to calm the nerves.

CHAYOTE

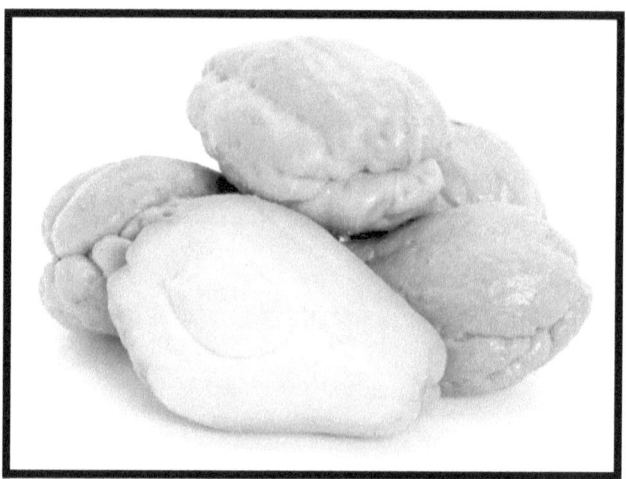

Chayote looks like a large pear, thus named vegetable pear or alligator pear. It belongs to the family of melons, cucumber, and squash. It is native to Latin America and is a popular ingredient in Mexican, Indian, and Latin American dishes. It has thin, green, wrinkly skin, a creamy dense texture, a mildly sweet taste similar to cucumber, and a flattened, white, single pit. Like tomato, chayote is actually a fruit that is used as a vegetable.

Chayote can be eaten raw, cooked, mashed, baked, boiled, and pickled. The root, stem, seeds, and young leaves are all edible.

Chayote is a good source of fibre, many amino acids, vitamins (C, B, and K), minerals (manganese, copper, zinc, magnesium, potassium, calcium, iron, phosphorus), and antioxidants (luteolin, apigenin).

Chayote protects the body from gaining weight, constipation, anaemia, infections, heart disease, stroke, birth defects, fatigue, abnormal blood clots, Alzheimer's disease, and free radicals.

Chayote lowers the risk of some cancers, premature ageing, osteoporosis, irritability, depression, and insomnia.

Tea made with chayote leaves is used to lower blood pressure, dissolve kidney stones, and treat the hardening of arteries.

Tea made from chayote flesh is a mild diuretic and is used in treating bloating.

CHICORY (POOR MAN'S COFFEE)

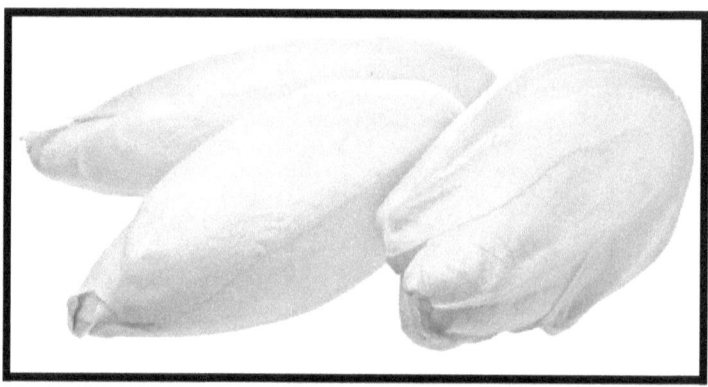

Chicory is a green, bitter, bushy herbal vegetable with light blue or lavender flower and a single, thick, white root. It is native to Europe, India, and Egypt. Chicory is one of the oldest-recorded types of plants. Each part of chicory has its uses: leaves are used as a salad vegetable, seed and flower extracts are used in traditional medicine and modern drug industry, and the root, after roasting and grinding, is used as a coffee substitute or added as an ingredient to coffee.

The key components of chicory are vitamins (K, C, A), minerals (potassium, calcium, phosphorus, copper, iron, manganese, magnesium), inulin, lactucin, hydroxycoumarins, flavonoids, protein, fibre, tannins in roots, and volatile oils in seeds.

Having no caffeine, it is a great substitute for coffee, thus lowering or eliminating dependence on caffeine.

Having the polysaccharide inulin, it regulates blood glucose level and lowers blood cholesterol and the risk of colon cancer, and it can be used as a plant-based sweetener.

It stimulates immune system.

It improves appetite.

It improves bile secretion and acts as a natural detoxifier.

It increases urine output and lowers kidney inflammation.

It stimulates bowel movement and acts as a laxative.

It regulates heartbeat.

It has anti-inflammatory effect and lowers swelling and pain of arthritis.

It neutralises stomach acidity and prevents acid reflux.

Lactucin acts as a sedative.

Extract from chicory leaf is used for the treatment of sore breasts in lactating mothers.

It encourages the growth of beneficial bacteria in the gut and thus promotes digestion and absorption of nutrients, an effect similar to the effect of beneficial bacteria in yogurt.

Collard Greens (Colewort)

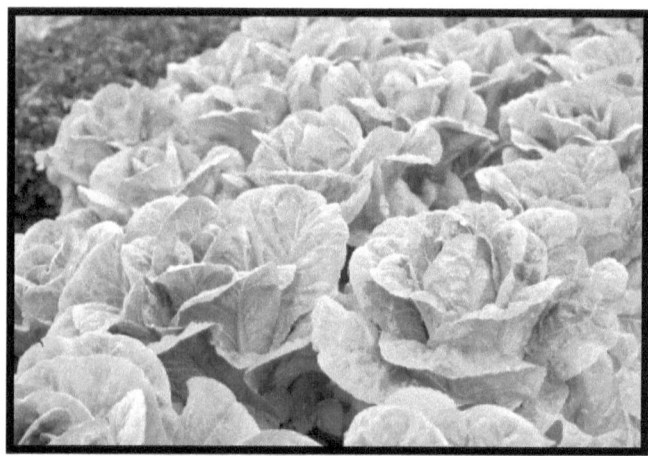

Collard greens belong to the brassica or mustard family and specifically to acephalea (headless) group. The name 'collard' is derived from *colewort*, meaning cabbage plant. Collard is a descendent of wild cabbage. It originated in the Mediterranean Basin and was a favourite food for ancient Romans and Greek. The leaves are dark green and broader than kale. It has a smooth, thick texture and a slightly bitter taste.

Collard is a rich source of fibre, vitamins (A, C, K, and folic acid), minerals (calcium, magnesium, potassium, and phosphorus), carotenoids (beta-carotene, lutein, zeaxanthin), and phytochemicals (indoles, sulphoraphane, and glucosinolates).

Indoles and sulphoraphane have benefits against several types of cancers (prostate, breast, cervical, ovarian, colon).

Vitamin C boosts immunity.

Fibre protects against constipation, haemorrhoids, and colon cancer.

Folic acid is involved in DNA synthesis and prevention of neural tube defect in newborns.

Vitamin A and carotenoids are essential for healthy vision, lung, skin, and oral cavity.

Vitamin K increases bone density, forms normal blood clots, and prevents against Alzheimer's disease.

CORN (MAIZE)

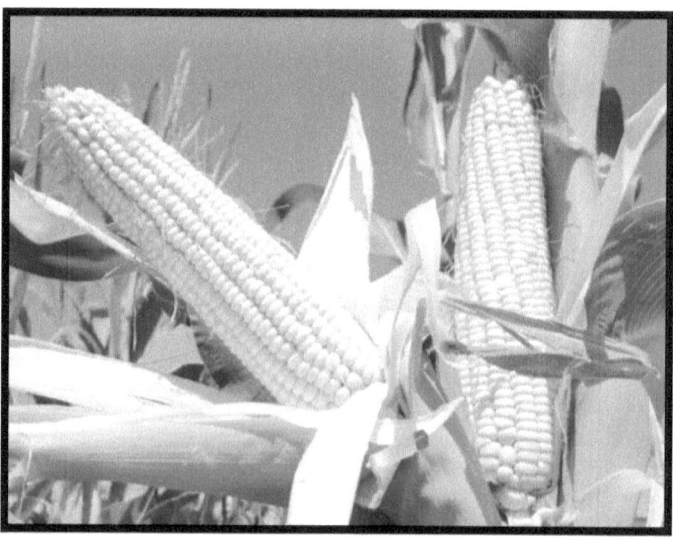

Corn originated in Mexico and Central America, where it has been food staple for over 7,000 years. Corn is one of the most popular cereals in the world and is the staple food in many countries. Although corn is a grain, its kernels are used in cooking as a vegetable. One ear of corn has 8-22 rows and contains around 800 kernels. The kernels are tender, juicy, and sweet. Although the kernels are usually yellow or white, they could be red, purple, blue, or brown.

Corn is a good source of fibre, vitamins (C, A, E, B1, B5, folic acid), minerals (phosphorus, manganese), carotenoids (beta-carotene, lutein, zeaxanthin, beta-cryptoxanthin), and the phenolic compound called ferulic acid.

Beta-cryptoxanthin lowers the risk of lung cancer.

Folic acid lowers blood homocysteine level, thus preventing heart diseases.

Fibre prevents constipation, haemorrhoids, and colorectal cancer.

Vitamins A, C, E, and manganese act as antioxidants.

Manganese and phosphorus aid in the formation of healthy bones.

Vitamin B-complex is important in energy production.

The caloric content (342 per 100 g) is among the highest in cereals.

Ferulic acid fights liver and breast cancers.

Carotenoids are important for healthy vision.

Anthocyanins in purple corn act as scavengers of cancer-causing free radicals.

CUCUMBER

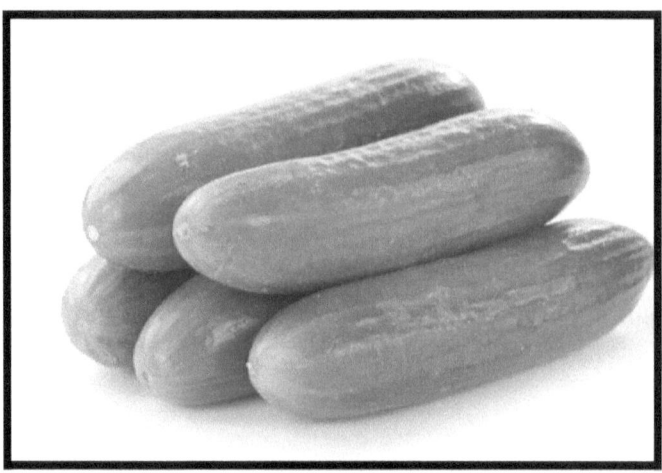

Cucumber belongs to the gourd family, which includes melons and squash. Botanically, cucumber is a fruit because it is a part of a flowering plant that comes from the ovary. Cucumber originated in India. Now, it is the fourth most cultivated vegetable in the world, after tomato, onion, and cabbage. There are two types of cucumbers, namely, slicing type and pickling type. The pickling variety is smaller and thicker and has bumpy skin with black-dotted spines.

Cucumber contains fibre, vitamins (K, C, and B5), minerals (molybdenum, potassium, manganese, magnesium, silicon, and sulphur), tryptophan, and phytochemicals (flavonoids, lignans, triterpenes).

The presence of lignans lowers the risk of breast, ovarian, uterine, and prostate cancers.

Low calorie and fat and high water (96%) and fibre aid in weight loss.

Potassium, magnesium, and fibre work synergistically to lower blood pressure.

Fibre and sterols lower blood cholesterol.

It is useful in type 2 diabetes.

Eating a cucumber a day will keep constipation away.

High water content makes it a natural diuretic.

Silicon strengthens the connective tissues and lowers the arthritic pain.

High water content, vitamins A, B, and C, potassium, and silica help with skin care.

Silica and sulphur stimulate healthy hair growth.

Electrolytes found in cucumber aid in hangover relief in some individuals.

Daikon (White Radish, Japanese Radish, Chinese Radish, Oriental Radish, Mooli)

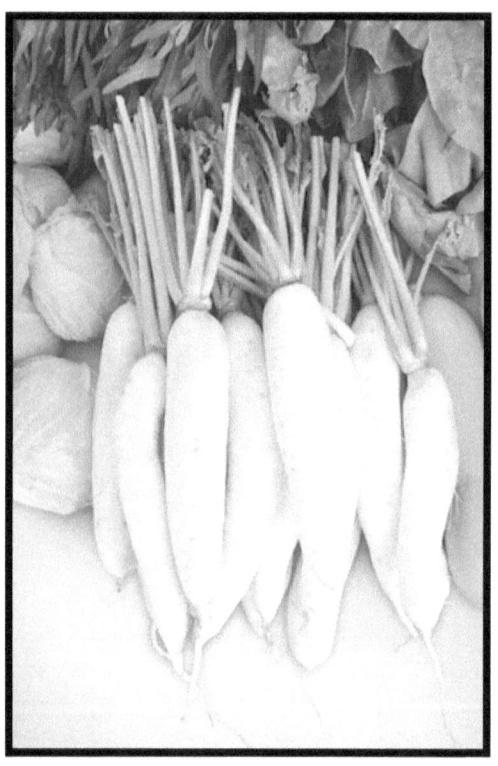

Daikon is a cruciferous root vegetable, related to broccoli, kale, and cabbage. It is a smooth, mild-flavoured giant root with a pungent, earthy smell. It originated in East Asia. Actually, daikon in Japanese means 'large root'. Daikon comes in many colours (usually white but also yellow, green, or black), shapes (spherical, oblong, and cylindrical), and sizes (it could weigh up to 45 Kg).

Daikon can be eaten raw, steamed, stir-fried, pickled or added to soups, and salads.

Daikon is a rich source of vitamins (C, B), minerals (potassium, calcium, iron, copper, sulphur, and phosphorus), fibre, enzymes, and phytochemicals (such as indoles).

It has anticancer properties.

It is a weight reducer and basal metabolic rate increaser.

It is cardioprotective.

It is a stroke preventer.

It is a diuretic and decongestant

It boosts immunity.

It is mucolytic.

It is a bone builder

It is a digestive.

It is a detoxifier

It is an anti-acne.

Dandelion Greens

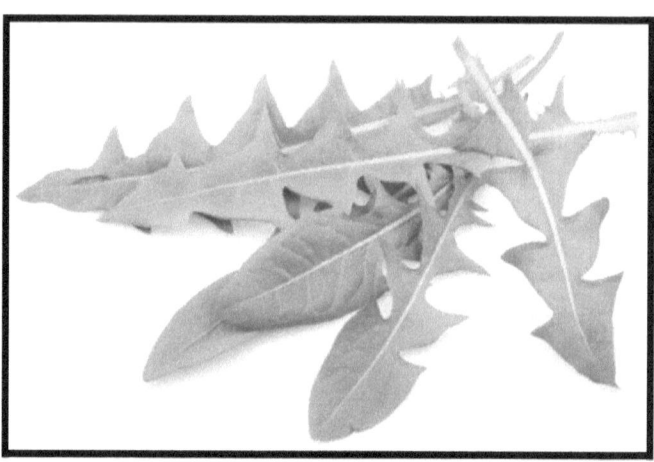

Dandelion greens have sharply serrated green leaves that resemble teeth, giving the plant its French name *Dent-de-Lion*, lion's teeth. The leaves grow in clusters. There is one pretty, yellow flower per stem, which turns into a white puffball after maturation. The root is fleshy, brown externally, containing bitter, milky latex internally. Leaves taste like chicory and endive with a bitter tinge and can be used in salads and smoothies. Flowers can be eaten raw or made into jams. Roots can be used for medicinal purposes or as coffee substitutes. Dandelion green originated in Central Asia and has been used for thousands of years in China, Europe, and the Americas for its medicinal properties.

It is a high source of complete protein, containing all the essential amino acids, fibre, vitamins (K, A, C, E, some B), minerals (calcium, manganese, iron, potassium, magnesium, phosphorus, copper), and carotenoids (alpha—and beta-carotenes, lutein, zeaxanthin, cryptoxanthin). It has more beta-carotene than carrots and more iron than spinach. Its vitamin K content is higher than all the herbs, providing 650% of required daily allowance.

The root contains inulin, which regulates blood sugar in diabetics.

Taracin triggers gall bladder and liver to release bile and stimulate the digestive system.

It is a natural diuretic, thus nicknamed *Piss-Lo-Lit*, meaning bed-wetter.

The root has antiviral properties.

It lowers the risk of breast and prostate cancers.

It contains two hormones (taraxerol and taraxasterol) that aid in the treatment of postmenopausal symptoms.

It aids in healthy vision.

It is anti-inflammatory.

It is a bone builder.

It is an Alzheimer's disease preventer.

It corrects anaemia.

CATSEAR

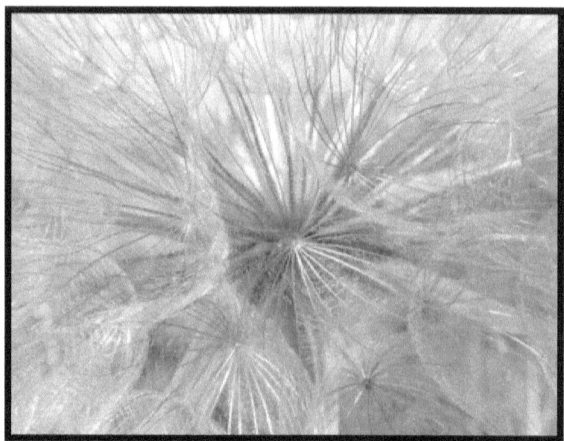

The catsear plant is native to Europe. Its leaves are similar to dandelion but have several branches coming from the same stalk, with a similar yellow flower, but unlike dandelion, it has hairy leaves. Catsear is derived from the words cat's ear and refers to the shape and fine hair on the leaves, resembling that of the ear of a cat.

The leaves can be eaten raw in salads, steamed or stir-fried. The roots may be roasted and used as coffee substitute.

Medicinal properties of catsear are similar to but less potent than dandelion.

EGGPLANT (AUBERGINE)

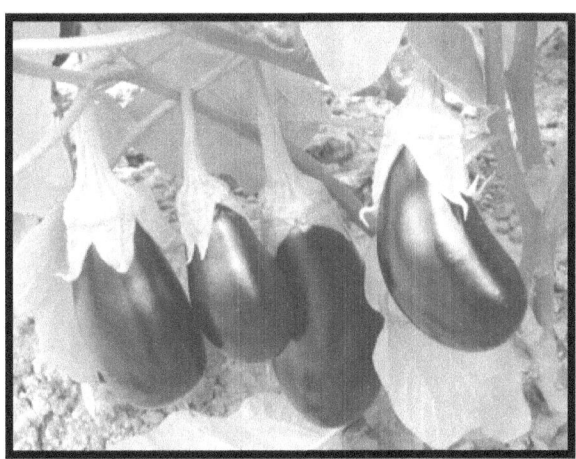

Eggplant originated in India as a wild plant. It was first cultivated in China, which is the world's top producer. Eggplant belongs to the nightshade family, which also includes tomato, potato and bell pepper. Eggplant most commonly has a deep purple colour, but it could come in white, yellow, orange, or reddish varieties as well. It has an oval, egg-like shape, hence the name. It has a pleasantly bitter taste and a spongy texture with numerous edible seeds.

Eggplant is a rich source of fibre, vitamins (C, K, B, and beta-carotene), minerals (manganese, molybdenum, potassium, and copper), tryptophan, and antioxidants, chlorogenic acid and nasunin.

Chlorogenic acid is the dominant antioxidant in eggplant. It fights free radicals, lowers blood cholesterol, inhibits cells from mutating into cancer cells, and has antiviral properties.

Nasunin is an anthocyanin found in the peels of eggplant, which has powerful antioxidant effect, preventing blood vessel formation (angiogenesis), thereby lowering the risk of cancer development. So eat your eggplant with its skin.

ENDIVE

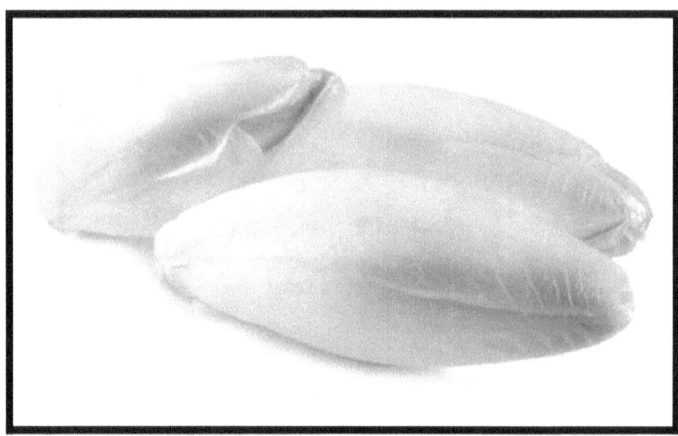

Endive is a green, leafy vegetable with a slightly bitter taste. It belongs to the daisy family of genus Cichorium and is closely related to chicory, radicchio, and dandelion. It looks like lettuce, but its leaves are curly and compressed into compact heads. The leaves are smooth and have cream colour. Endive has been in existence since ancient time and has been used by Greek, Romans, and Egyptians. Endive can be added to salads and soups, sautéed, or stewed.

Endive is a rich source of fibre, vitamins (A, B, C, E, and K), and minerals (manganese, copper, iron, potassium, magnesium, phosphorus, calcium, zinc).

Among all the vegetables, endive is one of the richest sources of vitamin A, important for healthy vision, skin, lungs, and oral cavity.

Its high vitamin E content helps to prevent Alzheimer's disease.

It lowers the risk of cancers of rectum, bladder, ovarian, and prostate cancers.

It is diuretic and laxative.

It is an appetiser, a bone builder, a blood former, and an Immunity booster.

Escarole

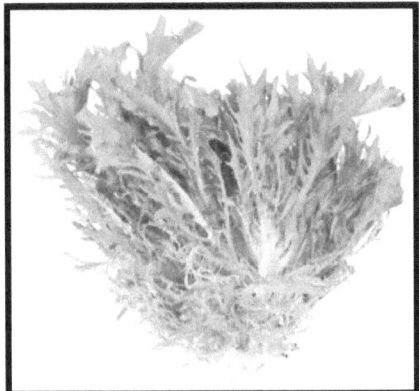

Escarole is a variety of endive whose leaves are broader, paler, and less bitter than other members of the endive family.

Fraiser (Curly Endive)

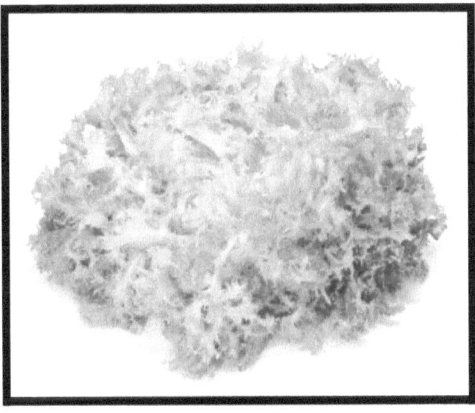

Fraiser is a member of the endive family with finely curled, attractive light-green or yellowish leaves that resemble feathered lettuce. It has a slightly bitter taste and is used in salads. It is very popular in France.

FENNEL

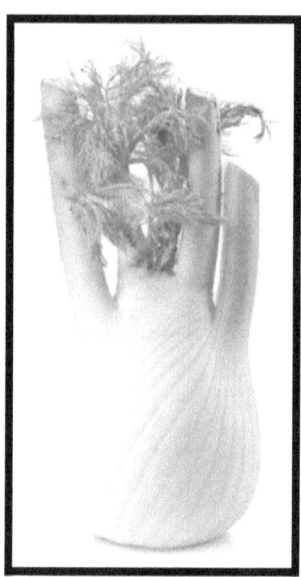

Fennel is composed of a white or light-green bulb, large green stalk, feathery leaves, and yellow flowers that produce grooved seeds. Fennel is highly aromatic with a crunchy texture like celery and sweet, anise-like taste. All parts of the plant, including bulb, stalk, flowers, and seeds, are edible. Fennel belongs to the same family as anise, cumin, parsley, dill, coriander, and carrot. It is indigenous to the Mediterranean region. Fennel can be eaten raw, sautéed, stewed, braised, or grilled.

Fennel is rich in fibre, vitamin C, folic acid, niacin, potassium, manganese, magnesium, phosphorus, calcium, iron, copper, and flavonoids (quercetin, rutin, kaempferol, glycosides).

Flavonoids act as antioxidants.

Anethole in the volatile oil has anti-inflammatory and anticancer properties.

It relieves heartburn, intestinal gas, bloating, colic in infants, and loss of appetite.

It treats cough and bronchitis by decreasing secretions.

It is a natural diuretic.

It increases breast milk flow.

It promotes menstruation.

It eases the birthing process.

It increases libido.

It improves hair quality.

Fennel oil is used as a flavouring agent.

Fennel oil is used in mouth freshness gargles, tooth pastes, antacids, and cough syrups.

FIDDLEHEAD

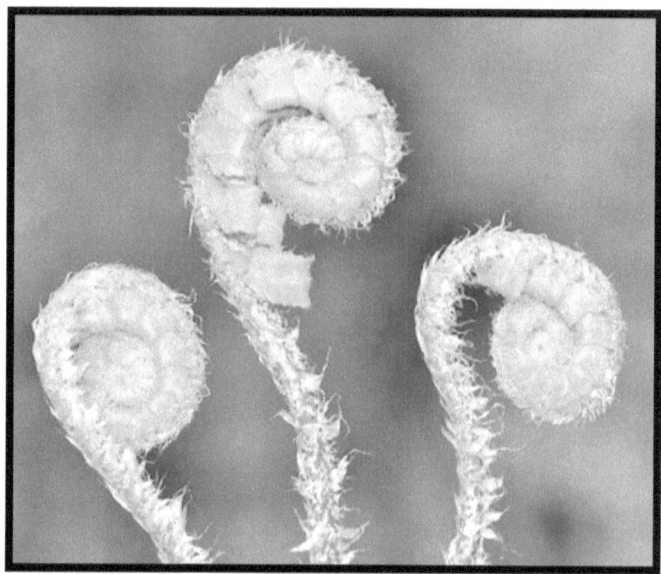

Fiddleheads are the curled tips of certain immature ferns that have not uncoiled yet. They are part of the traditional cuisines in France, Asia, and native Americas.

Fiddlehead greens are the premium wild forage with exquisite form and delicious flavour, a blend of artichoke, fava beans, and mushroom. Fiddlehead can be steamed, sautéed, or pickled but never eaten raw because it harbours toxins and bacteria and tastes bitter. Some varieties are also carcinogenic.

Fiddleheads are a good source of fibre, vitamin A, vitamin C, iron, potassium, antioxidants, and omega fatty acids.

GARLIC

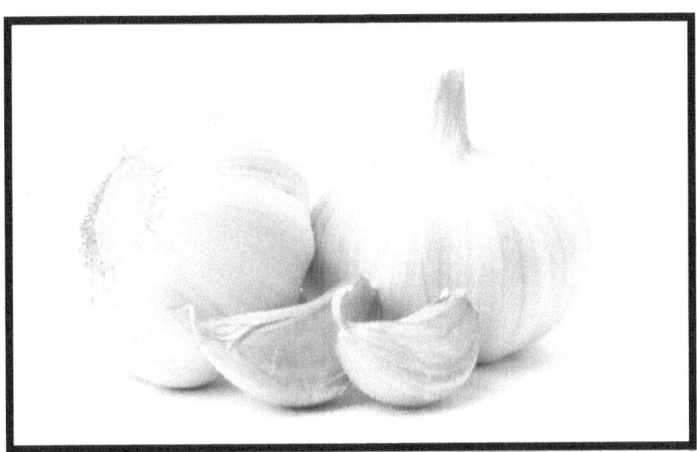

Garlic belongs to the allicin family that also includes onion, leek and chives. Garlic is native to Central Asia and has been used as a food and medicine in many cultures for thousands of years, dating back to when Egyptian pyramids were built.

There are more than 300 varieties of garlic available. Garlic has pungent, spicy taste, which sweetens with cooking. Each bulb is made up of four to twenty cloves, weighing about one gram each.

Garlic is a good source of fibre, vitamins (C, B6, and B1), minerals (manganese, calcium, phosphorus, copper, selenium), and the organic sulphur compound allicin.

Garlic is one of the most valuable super foods available to us.

It lowers the risk of colon and stomach cancers.

Garlic has the greatest antimicrobial activity of any vegetable we know. It is effective against cold and flu and bronchitis. It also acts as antiseptic, curing wounds.

Garlic has powerful antioxidant and anti-inflammatory activities due to the presence of vitamin C, copper, manganese, selenium, and sulphur compounds.

Garlic helps to regulate blood glucose level.

Garlic lowers cholesterol, blood pressure, and abnormal blood clots.

Garlic decreases arthritic pain resulting from inflammation.

Garlic detoxifies the body from heavy metals, like mercury and lead.

Good King Henry
(Poor Man's Asparagus)

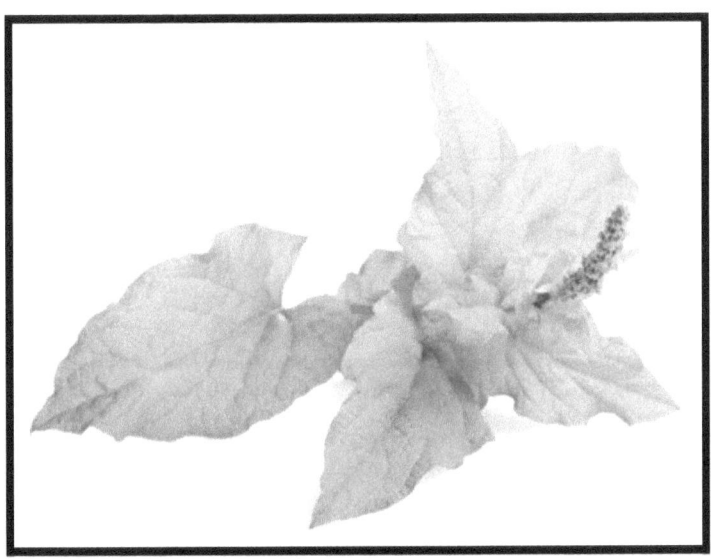

It is a species of goosefoot, native to Europe. It is considered a weed now.

It is a dark-green, succulent plant with large, thick, arrow-shaped leaves.

It is a delicious vegetable, which is eaten cooked like spinach or added to salads.

It is rich in fibre, vitamin C, vitamin A, calcium, and iron.

It is used as a digestive aid.

Green Beans (String Beans, Snap Beans)

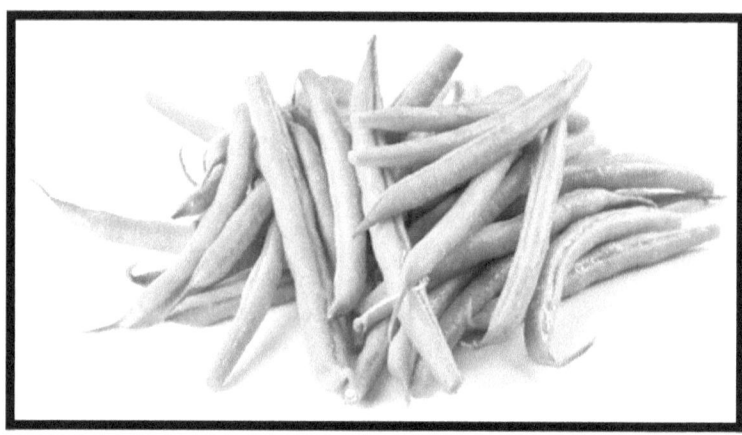

Green beans belong to the same family as shell beans, such as pinto beans, kidney beans, and fava beans. There are more than 300 varieties of green beans available. Green bean has a long, slender pod with small seeds inside. Although the most common colour is emerald green, it could come in golden, purple, red, or streaked varieties too.

Green bean is rich in fibre, vitamins (C, K, A, B), minerals (manganese, molybdenum, magnesium, potassium, iron, phosphorus, calcium, copper, zinc, silicon), tryptophan, protein, omega-3 fatty acids, carotenoids (beta-carotene, lutein, vidaxanthin, neoxanthin).

Green beans are one of the healthiest vegetables.

They are very low in calories and have low glycemic index, hence a great aid for diabetics and weight watchers.

They lower the risk of several cancers, such as breast and colon cancers.

They have powerful antioxidant and anti-inflammatory properties.

It is a cardioprotector and immune booster.

It is a bone builder

It aids in vision health

It helps in tissue builder and wound repair.

It is anti-depressive, and it nerve soother.

It is an Alzheimer's disease preventer.

GREEN PEAS

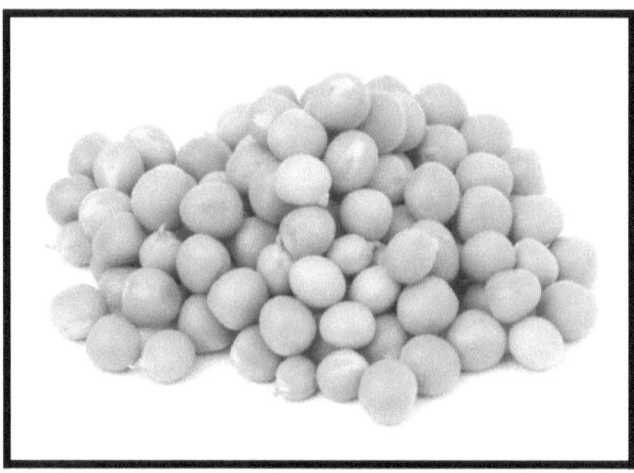

Pea is a legume belonging to the bean or pulse family, which also includes lentils, chickpeas, and dried beans. Legumes are plants that are in the form of pods, enclosing seeds known as beans. Pea pod is botanically a fruit because it contains seeds developed from the ovary of a flower, but it is consumed as a vegetable. There are up to five peas per pod. Three types of peas are available, namely, green or garden peas, snow peas, and snap peas. Although peas are most commonly green, there are purple and golden varieties.

Peas originated in the Mediterranean region, but it is now grown all over the world. Peas are hard but after boiling develop a mushy, tender texture and a sweet, starchy flavour.

Peas are a rich source of protein (one-quarter of the dry weight), fibre, vitamins (K, C, A, B), minerals (potassium, magnesium, calcium, phosphorus, manganese, iron, copper, zinc), omega-3 fatty acid, tryptophan, and phytochemicals (flavonols, phenolic acids, carotenoids, saponins, polyphenol coumestrol, phytosterols).

Phytosterol lowers blood cholesterol level.

Lectin is a protein that aids in dissolving blood clumps, preventing blood clot formation.

Coumestrol protects against stomach cancer.

High fibre and low calorie make it ideal to be included in the diet of diabetics and weight watchers.

It boosts Immunity and aids healthy vision.

It is a bone builder

It prevents Anaemia.

It is a cardioprotector.

It is anti-depressive and is nerve soother.

It is a tissue builder and wound healer.

HORSERADISH

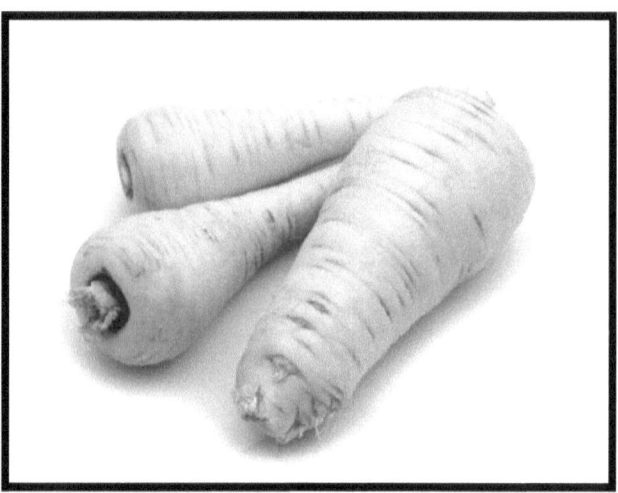

Horseradish is an ancient plant, native to South-East Europe and west India. It is cultivated for its large, white, tapered roots, which have a strong, hot, and sharp flavour and are used as condiment and medicine. Horseradish belongs to cabbage family, which also includes radish.

Horseradish is a rich source of fibre, vitamin C, potassium, calcium, magnesium, phosphorus, glucosinolates, and allyl isothiocyanates.

Glucosinolates increases the liver's ability to destroy carcinogens and suppress tumour growth, especially colorectal and lung cancers.

Horseradish contains mustard oil, which has antibacterial activity due to the presence of allyl isothiocyanates.

Its anti-inflammatory effects lower swelling and pain of arthritis and asthma attacks.

It is an expectorant and bronchodilator.

It is a coronary vasodilator, and it lowers blood pressure.

It stimulates appetite and digestion.

It is anti-parasitic.

It is a liver detoxifier.

It stimulates immune system.

It is a diuretic.

It is a sinus decongestant.

It soothes the nerve.

It is an aphrodisiac.

It can be used locally to remove spots and blemishes from the skin.

Jerusalem Artichoke
(Sunchoke, Sunroot, Earth Apple)

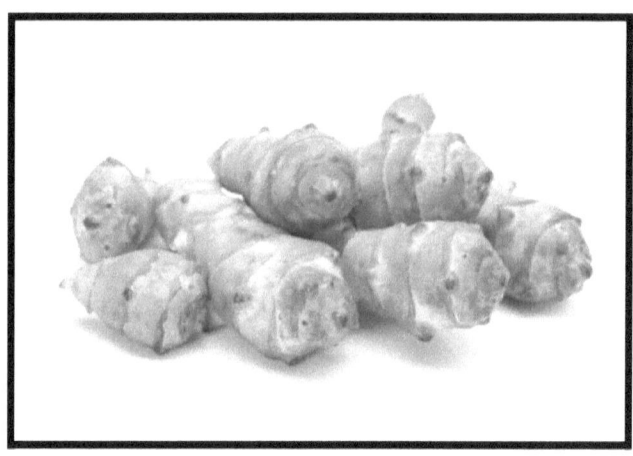

Sunchoke is a member of the sunflower family, native to North America. It is a bumpy, fleshy, nutty root like ginger and is eaten much the same way as potatoes and jicama. It varies in colour from white to brown, red, and purple. Despite its name, it has no relation to either Jerusalem or to artichoke. The taste resembles artichoke, but the plant is similar to sunflower.

Sunchoke can be eaten raw in salads, stir-fried, baked, steamed, pickled, or roasted. The tubers can be used as a substitute for potato, although it is sweeter and nuttier.

Sunchoke is a rich source of polysaccharide inulin, fibre, magnesium, phosphorus, potassium, iron, and some B vitamins.

Inulin is not utilised in the body for energy production; thus, it improves blood sugar control, making it useful for diabetics.

Inulin supports the beneficial bacteria in the gastrointestinal tract.

Jerusalem artichoke is cultivated for human consumption, alcohol production, and livestock feed and fructose production.

Jicama (Yam Bean)

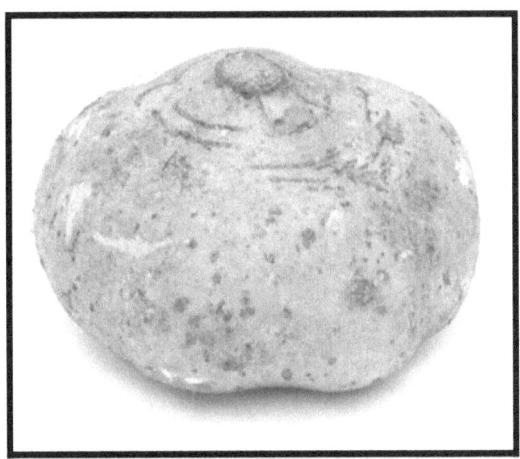

Jicama is a root vegetable belonging to the bean family. It resembles a large potato or brown turnip. It is related to sweet potato, but unlike potato and sweet potato, which can be eaten with their thin skin, jicama has a thick skin and must be peeled before eating. The flesh is ivory white, juicy, crunchy sweet, similar to water chestnut. Each tuber weighs 250 to 1,200 grams and contains inulin.

Inulin cannot be metabolised in the body and thus contributes no calories and is ideal as sweet snack for dieters and diabetics.

Jicama can be eaten raw, stir-fried, or baked.

Jicama is a good source of fibre, vitamin C, vitamin B6, potassium, magnesium, manganese, and copper.

Kai-lan
(Chinese Broccoli, Chinese kale)

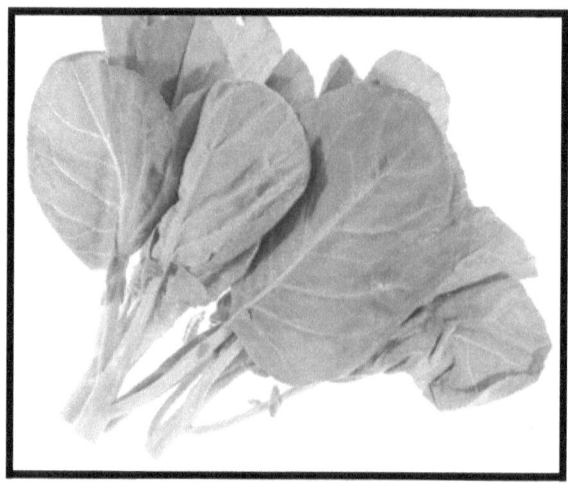

Kai-lan is a brassica vegetable, which also includes broccoli, Brussels sprouts, kale, and cauliflower. It has thick, flat, glossy, blue-green leaves, thick small stems, and a number of tiny green flower heads, similar to those of broccoli. The taste is similar to broccoli but stronger and slightly bitter.

Kai-lan is native to China and is popular in Asian cuisine. It is stir-fried, steamed, boiled, or added to soups. With broccoli, only the flower head is eaten, but with kai-lan, the leaves and stems are also eaten. Kai-lan is the most flavourous Chinese vegetable.

Kai-lan is a rich source of fibre, vitamins (A, C, K), and minerals (potassium, calcium, iron, manganese, copper, phosphorus).

Kale (Borecole)

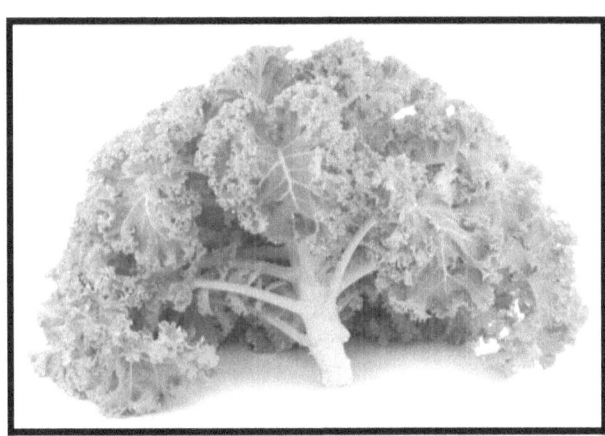

Kale belongs to the brassica family. It is a type of cabbage with green or purple leaves, in which the central leaves do not form a head. Kale has large, hardy, curly leaves, which are mildly bitter. Kale can be eaten raw, stir-fried, or added to soups.

Kale is a rich source of fibre, omega-3 fatty acids, vitamins (K, C, A), minerals (potassium, calcium, phosphorus, copper, iron, manganese), carotenoids (beta-carotene, lutein, zeaxanthin), and sulphur compounds (sulphoraphane, indoles).

Antioxidants, phytochemicals, and sulphur compounds lower the risk of bladder, breast, colon, ovary, and prostate cancers.

It is cardioprotective.

It is a liver detoxifier.

It enhances immune system.

It corrects Anaemia.

It is a bone builder.

It aids in vision health.

It prevents constipation.

It is anti-arthritic.

It is anti-asthma.

It prevents Alzheimer's disease.

Kohlrabi (German Turnip)

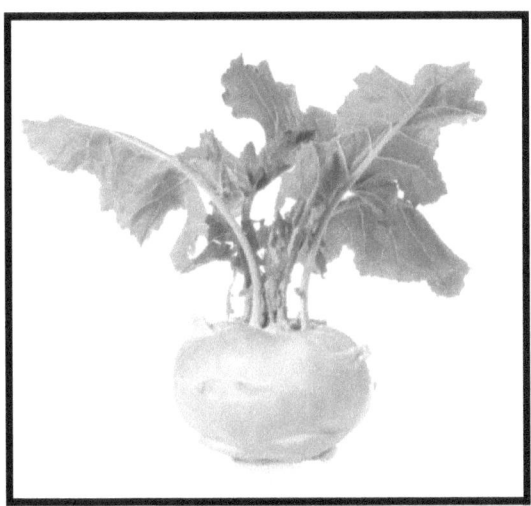

In German, kohlrabi means cabbage turnip. Its appearance is a cross between cabbage and turnip. Kohlrabi is of Eastern Europe origin. It belongs to the cabbage family. It is not a root vegetable but grows above the ground.

The globular, succulent stem of the plant is the part that is commonly eaten, but the large turnip-flavoured leaves are edible too and can be added to salads.

Kohlrabi is the size of an orange that has unique shape. It is similar in taste and texture to the broccoli stem or cabbage but is sweeter and milder. It can be white, light green, or deep purple with cream yellow flesh. The purple variety is spicier, but the other is sweeter.

Kohlrabi can be eaten raw, grilled, or stir-fried.

Kohlrabi is rich in fibre, vitamins (C, B, A), minerals (potassium, phosphorus, calcium, magnesium, iron, copper, manganese), omega fatty acids, and phytochemicals (isothiocyanates, sulphoraphane, indoles). Kohlrabi leaves are also rich in vitamins and minerals.

It protects against cancer.

It boosts Immunity.

It is a cardioprotector and bone builder.

It prevents anaemia.

It prevents constipation.

It aids in diet.

Komatsuna
(Japanese Mustard Spinach)

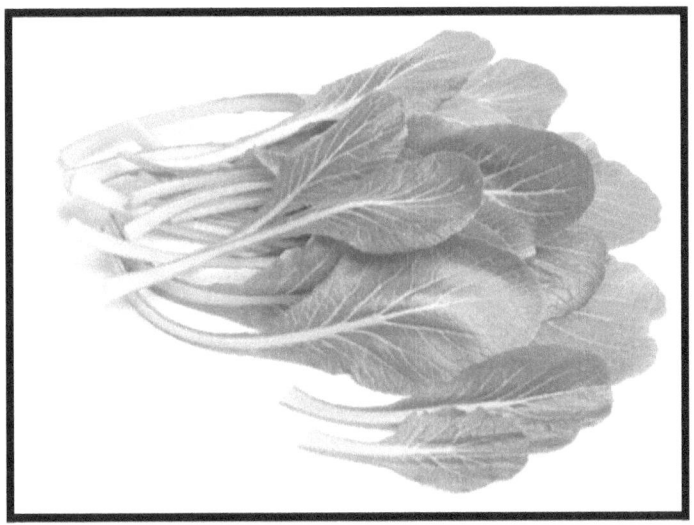

Komatsuna is a large, glossy, dark green leafy vegetable, which is a variant of turnip. It has thick, fleshy, light-green stalks. It is native to Japan, Korea, and Taiwan.

It is usually eaten stir-fried, boiled, pickled, or added to soups and salads. The young leaves, stalks, and flower shoots are all edible.

Komatsuna is similar to spinach in that it contains many important nutrients but is richer in iron, is delicious, and does have bitterness of spinach.

Komatsuna is low in calories, but it is a rich source of vitamin C, vitamin A, and calcium. It also has some fibre, protein, vitamin K, and potassium.

Lamb's Quarters (Wild Spinach, Pigweed, Fat-Hen, Goosefoot)

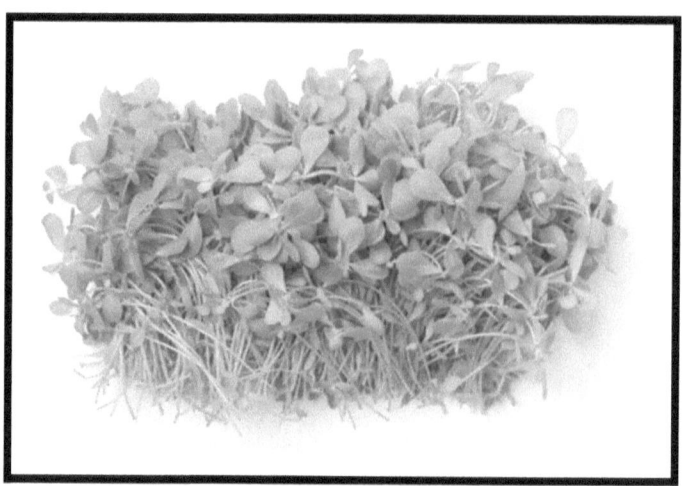

It is a common weed with edible stem and leaves that grow wild throughout the world. Its use dates back to Native Americans.

It resembles the webbed feet of geese, hence the name goosefoot. It is a relative of chard, beets, and orach.

The stems have red stalks. The leaves are either triangular or diamond-shaped, have few 'teeth' in the edges, and are white underneath. The flavour is similar to spinach or chard with an earthy metallic taste. It is eaten as salad or cooked.

It is the second highest nutritious of all wild weeds after amaranth.

It is rich in vitamins (K, A, C, B) and minerals (manganese, calcium, iron, magnesium, phosphorus, potassium, copper, zinc).

Lamb's quarters contain oxalic acid and must be avoided by those who have kidney stone or kidney disease.

LEEKS

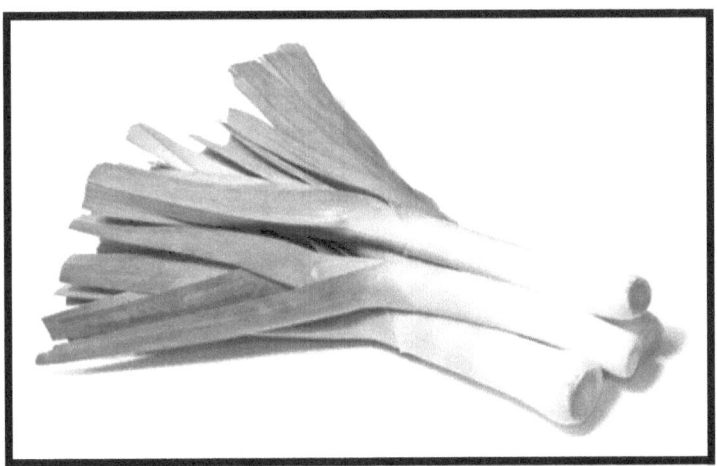

Leeks belong to the allium family, which includes onions and garlic, but unlike others, leeks do not form bulbs. Leeks look like scallions but are firmer and denser. The edible part of the leeks is a long cylinder of bundled leaf sheaths, called stem or stalk. The flavour of leeks is milder and sweeter than that of onion.

Leeks were cultivated in the Mediterranean region thousands of years ago.

Leeks are a good source of fibre, vitamins (A, C, K, and folic acid), minerals (calcium, magnesium, phosphorus, potassium iron, and manganese), carotenoids (lutein, beta-carotene, zeaxanthin), and organosulphur compounds.

These sulphur compounds convert to allicin in the body, where they perform several functions as follows:

+ They lower cholesterol synthesis in the liver.
+ They decrease the stiffness of blood vessels by releasing nitric oxide and thus lowering blood pressure.
+ They prevent blood clot formation, thus lowering the risk of heart attack and stroke.

Benefits of eating leeks include the following:

- Cardioprotection
- Healthy vision
- Lowering of the risk of colon and breast cancers
- Antibacterial activity
- Bone builder
- DNA synthesis
- Weight reduction

Lettuce (King of Salads)

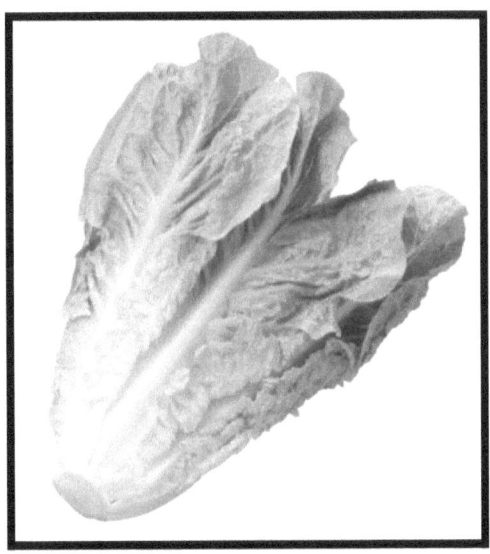

Lettuce belongs to the daisy family of Asteraceae. Lettuce derives its name from 'latex', referring to the plant's milky juice. Lettuce originated in the Mediterranean region and India, but today, it is grown all over the world. Lettuce is one of the most consumed vegetables in the world.

Lettuce is either green or crimson-red. It comes in hundreds of varieties, like butterhead, crisphead (iceberg), and leaf or romaine (cos). The classification is based on head formation and leaf structure.

Lettuce is a good source of fibre, vitamins (A, K, C, and B), minerals (manganese, iron, potassium, calcium, magnesium, phosphorus, copper, zinc, and molybdenum), carotenoids (beta-carotene, lutein, and zeaxanthin), phytochemicals (coumarins, flavonoids, and lactucin), and tryptophan and omega-3 fatty acids.

Lettuce is one of the low-calorie vegetables (15 calories/100 g) and thus aids in dieting.

It aids in digestion, cures constipation, and removes flatulence.

It lowers the risk of heart disease and stroke by decreasing blood cholesterol level, improving circulation and preventing atherosclerosis.

It lowers the risk of night blindness, cataract, and macular degeneration.

It lowers the risk of several types of cancers by its high content of phytochemicals and antioxidants.

Lactucarium in lettuce has the ability to induce sleep, calms the nerves, and controls palpitation.

It lowers the risk of anaemia.

It is a mild diuretic.

Celtuce

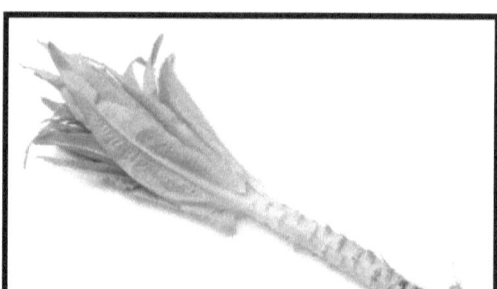

Celtuce, also known as Chinese lettuce, stem lettuce, celery lettuce, and asparagus lettuce, is a variety of lettuce that originated in southern China. It is named after the combination of celery-like stem and lettuce-like leaves.

In China, it is grown primarily for its fat, crispy, tender stalk. The large leaves have a mild celery-like flavour and can be used as lettuce in salads and stir-fries.

Lotus Root (Renken in Japanese)

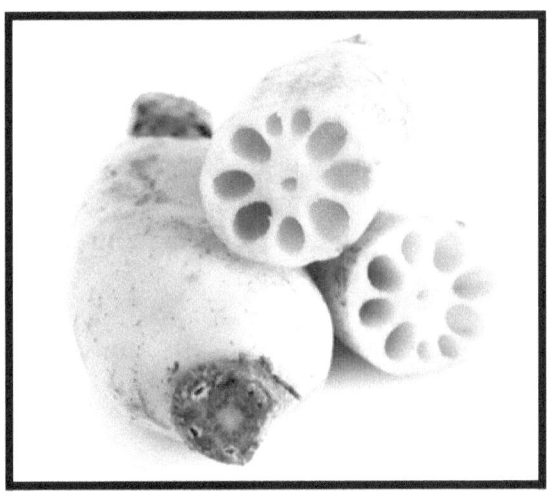

Lotus root is actually the rhizome of the lotus plant that grows under the water in the mud. It is indigenous to Asia. Lotus root is a starchy vegetable, like potato, with a reddish-brown skin and white, crunchy, mildly sweet flesh, tasting like artichoke or water chestnut.

In cross-section, symmetrical air canals (holes) appear, giving it an appealing look. Its shape looks like a long squash, the length of which could reach up to four feet. Even the seeds, petals, and leaves of the lotus plant are edible. Lotus root can be eaten raw, steamed, stir-fried, or candied.

Lotus flower represents purity, beauty, fertility, prosperity, spirituality, and eternity in Asian cultures.

In India, lotus flower is the national logo.

Lotus root is a rich source of fibre, vitamins C and B6, manganese, copper, iron, potassium, phosphorus, magnesium, and calcium.

Fibre helps lower cholesterol, glucose, and weight and prevents constipation.

Vitamin C is an excellent antioxidant, is involved in collagen synthesis and wound healing, and boosts immunity.

Vitamin B6 is used as a coenzyme in the neurochemical synthesis, which influences mood.

Potassium regulates blood pressure and heart rate.

Iron and copper are involved in red blood cell production.

Calcium, phosphorus, magnesium, and manganese function in building strong bones and preventing osteoporosis.

LUFFA

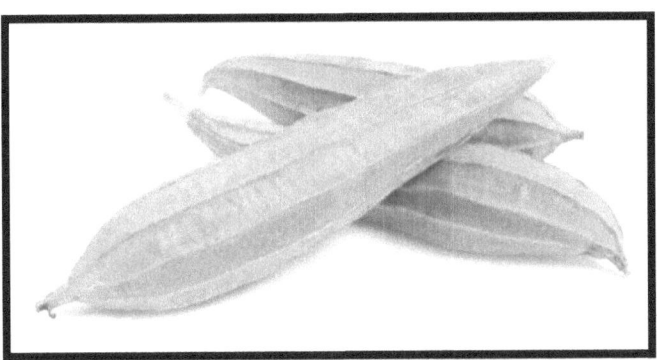

Luffa has many names, such as ridge gourd, dishcloth gourd, and vegetable sponge. It is native of the Asian tropics. It resembles a cucumber, but unlike cucumber, it forms a fibrous sponge after maturity. Thus, luffa fruit is edible only when immature.

Luffa is a dark-green ridged vegetable having white pulp and white seeds. The young fruit can be eaten raw like a cucumber or cooked like a squash.

Luffa has fibre, vitamin C, some B vitamins, iron, magnesium, calcium, phosphorus, and zinc.

Luffa contains insulin-like peptides, alkaloids, and charantin, which lower blood and urine glucose.

Luffa is a blood purifier, protecting liver from alcohol intoxication. Thus, its juice is used for the treatment of jaundice.

It is used to treat sinus problems.

It is used to relieve menstrual symptoms.

It is used to prevent breast milk production.

Luffa sponge exfoliates dead skin and enhances surface circulation.

Mache (Lamb's Lettuce, Corn Salad)

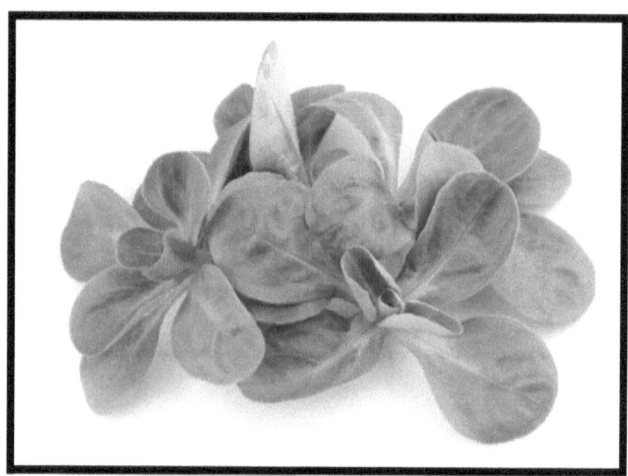

Mache is native to France, where it has been cultivated since the seventeenth century under the name *doucette*. It grows now in many parts of the world, including Europe, North Africa, and Western Asia.

Mache is one of the most delicate of salad greens. It forms a loose and waxy rosette of six to eight rounded, green, velvety leaves with a melting quality. The flavour is sweet, creamy, and nutty. The stems are lemon-lime in colour, tender, and succulent.

Mache is rich in fibre, protein, omega-3 fatty acids, carotenoids (beta-carotene, lutein, and zeaxanthin), vitamins (B, C), and minerals (calcium, phosphorus potassium, iron).

The high content of phytonutrients and antioxidants give mache anticancer and cardioprotective properties.

Malabar Gourd (Fig-Leaved Gourd, Asian Pumpkin, Pie Melon)

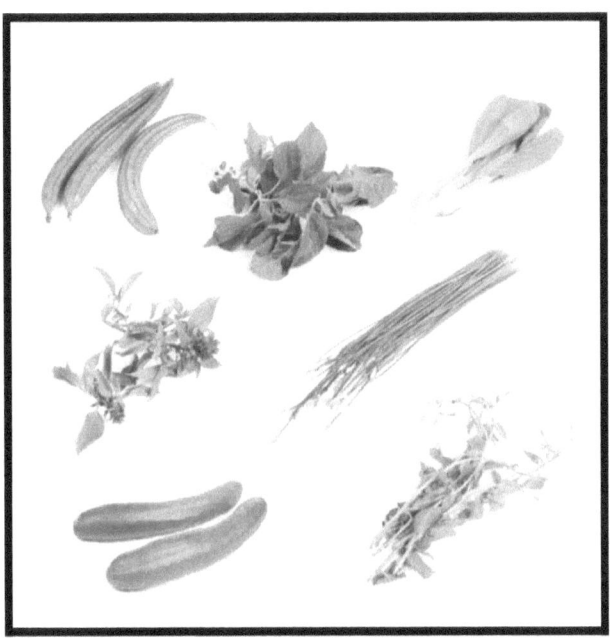

It is native to Americas, and it is very popular in Latin America. It is a member of the cucumber and melon family. It is a fairly large fruit, weighing as much as six kilograms.

The immature fruit can be consumed as a vegetable. Both the flowers and young shoots are eaten as leafy greens. The protein-rich and oil-rich seeds are also edible.

The fruit is bright green to dark green to cream in colour and oblong in shape and looks like a speckled or mottled watermelon. The leaves look like a fig; hence, the name fig-leaved gourd is given to it. The flowers are yellow to orange and contain as much as 500 seeds.

Malabar gourd is low in carbohydrates and calories and thus is an ideal diet food.

Malanga (Japanese Potatoes)

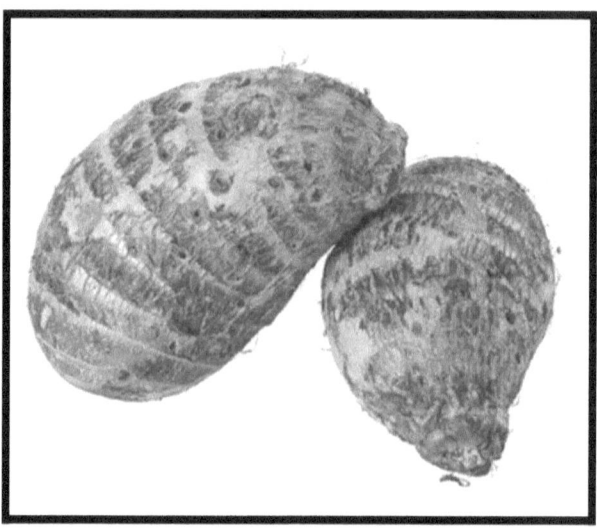

Malanga is a root vegetable that is a staple food in the West Indies and all the tropical, Spanish-speaking countries. It is a common ingredient in Cuban cuisine. Malanga flour is used as a substitute for wheat to make breads, cookies, muffins, pancakes, and chips. It can be used in soups and stews, and it is also used as a thickener.

Malanga root has a tough, irregular, brown, thin skin and could weigh up to two pounds.

The flesh is crispy white, yellow, orange, pink, or red. It resembles taro with large green leaves. Its consistency is similar to potato or sweet potato. The taste is strong and resembles hazelnut. The leaves are prepared like spinach but contain oxalates, whose bitter irritable taste can be neutralised by cooking.

Malanga is a rich source of fibre (10%), vitamins (C, B1, B2), and minerals (iron, phosphorus).

It is high in energy (135 calories per half a cup), thus beneficial for underweight and undernourished individuals.

It is free of gluten, which could cause abdominal pain and gas in intolerant individuals.

It is the most hypoallergenic food because its starch grains are the smallest and most easily digested of all the complex carbohydrates.

MALLOW

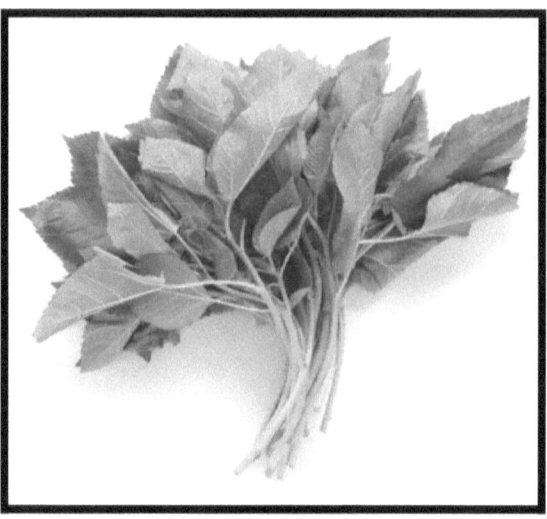

Mallow is grown wild in the Middle East, where it is known as *khubeza* in Arabic. It has bright, heart-shaped, curly-edged green leaves, slimy texture, and a mild lettuce taste. It is used as a main ingredient in Arab dishes and as a garnish to many Arabic dishes, soups, and stir-fries. The young leaves are mild and used as a substitute for lettuce. Older leaves are cooked as a leafy green vegetable. The buds and flowers can be used in salads.

The mallows represent a large group of flowering plants, including marshmallow, okra, rose mallow, jute, and cocoa and kola nut. A number of mallows are edible and have medicinal properties.

Mallow is one of the earliest plants cited in history. It is high in mucilage and acts as a thickening agent.

Mallow is rich in fibre, vitamin A, vitamin C, calcium, magnesium, potassium, iron, and selenium.

Mallow is a good digestive aid and coats and soothes the irritated mucous membranes due to the presence of mucilage.

Mallow is anti-inflammatory and is used in the treatment of sore gums, sore throats, and aches and pains.

Mallow is anti-tussive and is used in the treatment of cough.

Mallow soothes skin irritations.

Mashua

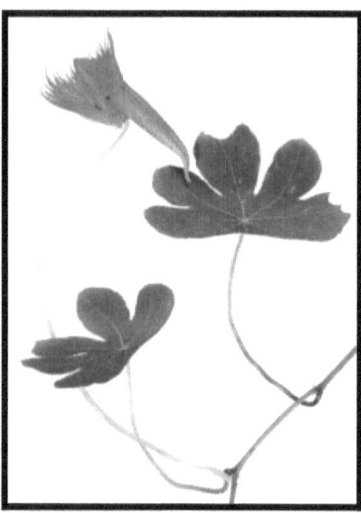

Mashua is a root vegetable that is a major food source in Andes regions of South America. The tubers or rhizomes are the size of small potatoes, and the shape ranges from conical to carrot-like. The tubers are white, yellow, red, or purple. The taste is peppery, like radish, due to the presence of isothiocyanates (mustard oil) but sweetens after boiling. It is used in soups, stir-fried, or baked. The flowers and young leaves are also edible.

Mashua is rich in a protein that contains all the essential amino acids, fibre, vitamin C, and beta-carotene.

It prevents stomach, colon, and prostate and skin cancers.

It is a diuretic.

It treats skin ulcers.

It is a remedy for certain kidney ailments.

It lowers libido and sex drive. It is a great tool to use for armies to forget their wives. So understandably, men should avoid it.

MOLOKHIA (EGYPTIAN'S SPINACH, JEW'S MALLOW)

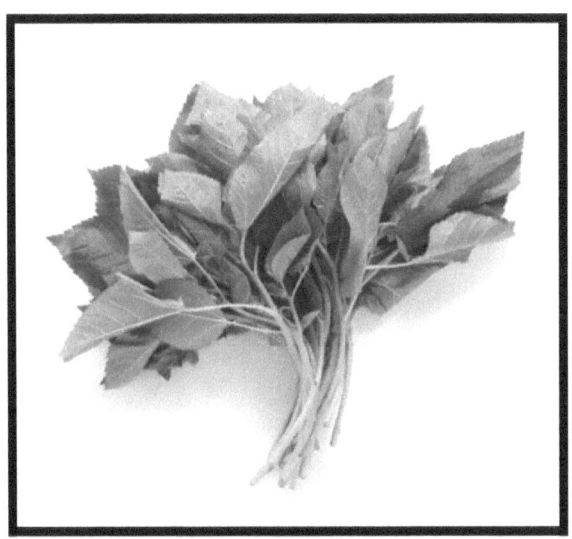

Molokhia is a dark-green, viscous, slimy, bitter leafy vegetable, similar in appearance to spinach. It originated in Egypt, where it is the national dish. Its use dates back to the Egyptian's Pharaohs. It was the favourite dish of Pharaohs, who ate it with rabbit. It was banned by the puritan Fatimid for its aphrodisiac effect, increasing the sexual desire. It is now a very popular vegetable in the Middle East.

Molokhia is also called Jew's mallow from a claim that Jewish priests discovered it.

Molokhia is not eaten raw but cooked as stew or soup.

Molokhia is a good source of fibre, vitamins (C, A, K, E), and minerals (calcium, manganese, iron, selenium, magnesium, potassium).

It increases blood flow. This could be the reason for its claimed aphrodisiac effect.

It has potent antioxidant and anti-inflammatory properties, preventing certain types of cancer, hardening of arteries, arthritis, and asthma.

It has a potent anti-ageing effect, so much so that Cleopatra's beauty is attributed to her consumption of this vegetable.

MORINGA (THE MIRACLE TREE)

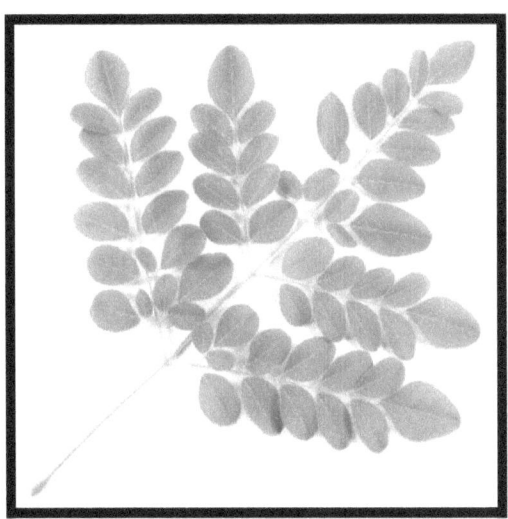

Moringa is the sole genus in the flowering plant family Mringacae, native to the Himalayas in north-western India. It has a history of thousands of years and has been recovered from the tombs of ancient Egyptians. It is now cultivated throughout the tropics.

Moringa is a universal plant, meaning, all its parts, including leaves, flowers, seeds, seed oil, roots and buds, are utilised.

Moringa is called drumstick tree because its seeds are slender, long, and triangular. It is also called horseradish tree because its roots taste like horseradish.

Moringa leaves are the most nutritious part of the plant, as they are rich in fibre, vitamin C, beta-carotene, calcium, potassium, magnesium, iron, protein, and phytochemicals. The leaves are eaten raw or fried.

Moringa seeds have 30 to 40% oil, mostly oleic acid. It also contains minerals and vitamins. The seeds are roasted like nuts.

MUSHROOM

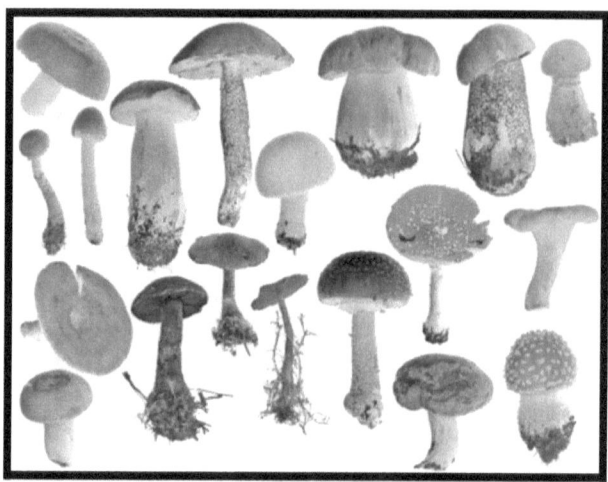

Mushrooms are classified as vegetables or herbs although they are not plants but fungi. They are saprophytes, without chlorophyll, that live by extracting nutrients from decaying plants or dead animal matters.

Mushrooms have been used as a food and medicine for thousands of years. The ancient Egyptians used it as delicacies, Greeks as energy boosters, Romans for feast, and Chinese for medicine.

There are more than 14,000 types of mushrooms, but only 3,000 varieties are edible, and less than 1% are poisonous. They vary in colour, texture, shape, and properties.

Mushrooms are added to soups, salads, sandwiches, and stews.

Mushrooms are rich in fibre, protein, vitamins (B, A, D), minerals (copper, selenium, potassium), and phytochemical antioxidants (ergothionene, beta-glucans, lentinan).

Mushroom is the only vegetable that contains vitamin D in edible form.

Mushroom is the best choice to obtain selenium from vegetables.

Lentinan is a glucan polysaccharide that increases the production of interleukin, a hormone that stimulates the immune system against infectious agents. It also improves the quality of life in patients who have undergone chemotherapy.

Beta-glucans inhibit cancerous cells of prostate, stimulates immune system against allergies, and participates in physiological processes related to the metabolism of fats and carbohydrates.

Ergothionene has strong antioxidant properties and reduces the risk of developing chronic diseases. Mushrooms contain much more of this compound than is found in wheat germ and chicken liver.

Conjugated linoleic acid suppresses the effect of oestrogen, which is responsible for breast cancer in postmenopausal women.

Mustard Greens (Indian Mustard, Chinese Mustard, Leaf Mustard)

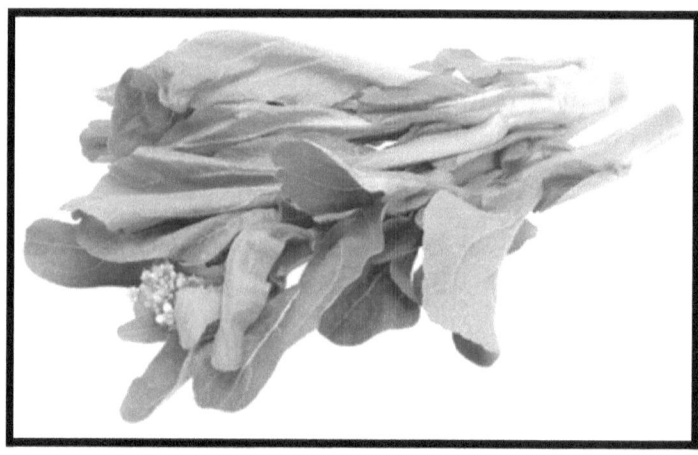

Mustard greens belong to the cabbage family. It has spicy, crunchy, pungent peppery leaves. It originated in the Himalayan region of India more than 5,000 years ago. Nowadays, they are mostly produced in South-East Asia for the leaves and for the production of oil seeds. Leaves, seeds, and stems are all edible. They produce seeds that are used to make mustard, hence the name mustard greens.

There are many varieties of mustard greens, mostly emerald green, but some are burgundy or deep purple.

Mustard greens are high in vitamins (K, A, C, B, E), minerals (manganese, calcium, potassium, phosphorus, iron, copper, magnesium), fibre, protein, tryptophan, omega-3 fatty acids, and phytochemicals (quercetin, hydroxycinnamic acid, isorhamnetin, kaempferol).

Being a rich source of antioxidants (vitamins C and E, manganese, flavonoids, carotenoids, indoles, sulphoraphane), mustard greens lower the risk of several cancers, such as breast, bladder, colon, lung, prostate, and ovarian cancers.

Being an excellent source of vitamin K and omega-3 fatty acids, the two powerful anti-inflammatory agents, mustard greens lower the severity of arthritic pain and asthma.

Benefits of mustard greens include the following:

- Cardioprotection
- Bone building
- Eye health
- Detoxification
- Weight reduction

OCA

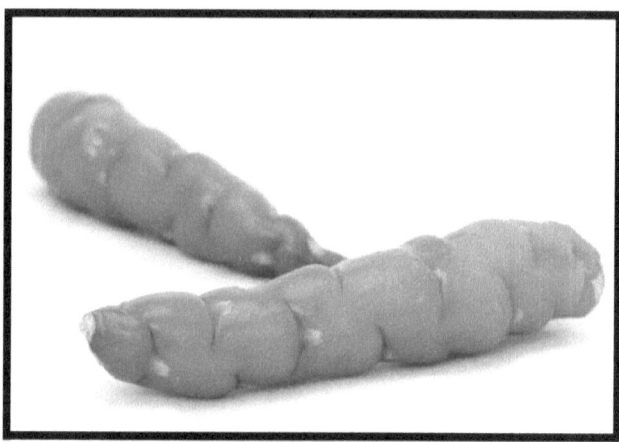

Oca is a long cylindrical tuber that originated in Andes region of South America, where it is the second most cultivated tuber after potato.

The colour varies from creamy white to pink, red, and purple. The flesh is white. The texture is crunchy like carrot when undercooked but becomes starchy when fully cooked. It has lemony flavour. The leaves can be eaten as a vegetable.

Oca can be eaten boiled, baked, roasted, fried, steamed, or added to soups.

Oca tubers and leaves contain oxalic acid, hence its scientific name Oxalis tuberosa.

Oca is rich in protein, fibre, carotenoids, vitamins C and B, iron, calcium, and potassium.

OKRA (LADY'S FINGER, GUMBO)

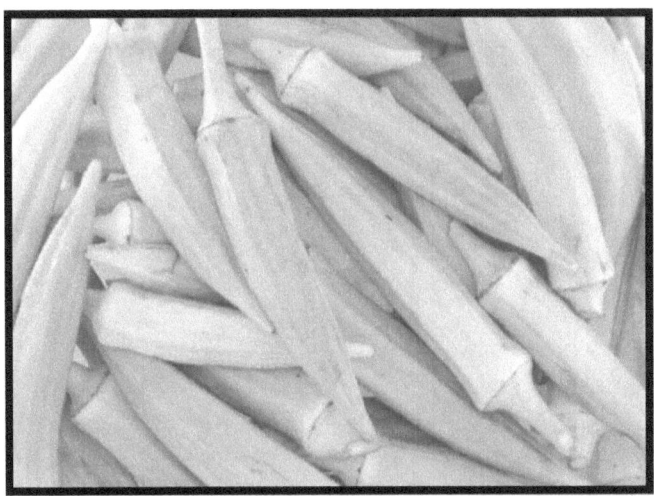

Okra is a flowering plant in the mallow family. It is of African origin, and Egyptians were the first to cultivate it. Okra is a highly nutritious green pod vegetable with finger-like curved pods. The pods have small, round, white mucilaginous seeds arranged in vertical rows. Okra can be eaten raw, stewed, fried, pickled, and braised.

Okra is a rich source of fibre, vitamins (C, K, B), minerals (manganese, magnesium, calcium, potassium, phosphorus, copper), and carotenoids (lutein, zeaxanthin, beta-carotene). Okra seeds contain protein and edible oil.

The slimy mucilage binds to cholesterol, bile acids, and toxins and inhibits their absorption.

The rich fibre and mucilage help in smooth peristalsis of digested food, prevent and treat constipation, lower the risk of colorectal cancer, and stabilise blood glucose level.

Okra propagates good bacteria in the intestine that assist in digestion.

Okra is a diuretic and is useful in treating cystitis (inflammation of bladder).

Because of high content of folic acid and B6, okra is an ideal vegetable during pregnancy.

Being low in calories and fat, okra is a great tool for losing weight.

Okra alleviates irritation, pain, and swelling in the throat, associated with flu.

Other benefits of okra include:

- Healthy vision
- Healthy bone
- Normal blood clot
- Immunity boosting

ONIONS

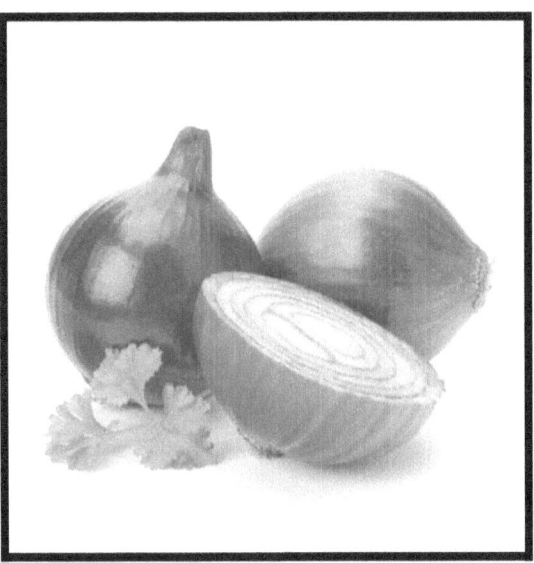

Can you imagine life without onion? I certainly cannot. I love to include it in every food I eat, whether it is stew, salad, soup, sandwiches, omelette, pickles, etc. Onions are the most produced crop in the world after tomato. Onion belongs to the allium family of root vegetables, which also includes garlic, leek, and chives.

Onions have been used for over 5,000 years by many cultures around the world. Onions are native to Asia and the Middle East. Ancient Egyptians used onion as gifts and for paying rent or salary. They worshipped onion and took it with themselves to their graves.

There are more than 600 varieties of onions, which come in different colours as white, red, yellow and green, each having a unique taste from mildly sweet to pungent.

Onions are rich sources of fibre, vitamins (C, K, B1, B6, B9), minerals (chromium, manganese, molybdenum, potassium, copper, phosphorus), quercetin, phenolic acids, sterols, saponins, volatile oils, tryptophan, and organosulphur compounds responsible for their pungent odour and for irritating the eyes. Quercetin in onions is the highest among all the vegetables, but the white variety is devoid of it. Onions also contain the enzyme allinase, which is released when onion is chopped, causing eyes to lacrimate. Although onion is rich in sulphur compounds, it is only one-fourth the level found in garlic.

Quercetin and sulphur compounds lower the risk of colon, stomach, head, and neck cancers.

The volatile organosulphur compounds compete with insulin for breakdown sites in the liver, thus increasing the lifespan of insulin. Chromium in onions improves cell's ability to respond to insulin.

Sulphur compounds detoxify the body from heavy metals.

Onions act as a natural food preservative and destroy many disease-causing pathogens. Onions are useful in oral health, fighting oral pathogens and dental decay.

Tryptophan is converted to neurotransmitters, which act as sedative and fight insomnia.

Onion increases digestive juices and is an appetiser.

Quercetin lowers the severity of arthritic pain.

Quercetin inhibits the production of compounds that cause the bronchial muscles to spasm and cause asthma attacks.

Folic acid and vitamin B6 decrease homocysteine level in the blood, which is a risk factor for heart attack and stroke.

It has been claimed that daily consumption of onion helps libido and premature ejaculation.

PARSLEY

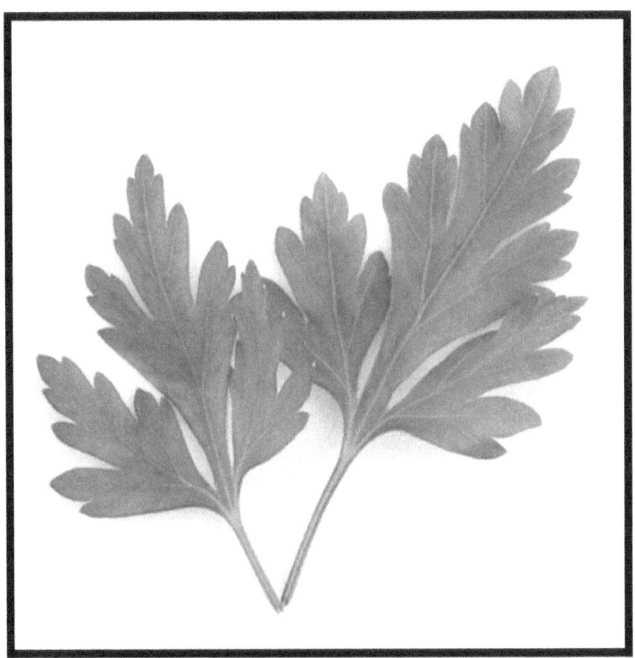

Parsley is native to the Mediterranean zone, where it is cultivated as a herb, a spice, and a vegetable. Parsley is a relative of celery. It has bright-green curly or flat leaf and a slightly bitter taste. The flat-leaved variety has a stronger flavour. Root parsley is used as a vegetable in stews, soups, and casseroles in Europe. Curly leaved variety is used as a garnish.

Parsley is a rich source of fibre, vitamins (folic acid, C, A, K), minerals (iron, calcium, potassium, magnesium, manganese, copper, zinc), luteolin, and essential oil.

Myristicin, an organic compound in the essential oil of parsley, inhibits tumour growth, especially in the lungs.

Luteolin is an antioxidant that eradicates the harmful free radicals. The presence of vitamins A and C and manganese also adds to parsley's antioxidant power.

Luteolin and vitamin C combat inflammatory diseases like arthritis and asthma.

Eugenol is an essential oil in parsley that is used as a local anaesthetic and antiseptic agent for teeth and gum diseases.

Vitamin K is necessary for the synthesis of osteocalcin, a protein that strengthens the composition of bones, and for the synthesis of sphingolipids that maintain myelin sheath around the nerves.

Folic acid converts the harmful homocysteine into harmless molecules and thus wards off heart attack and stroke.

Vitamins C and A strengthen immune system.

Parsley aids in digestion and imparts delicious flavour to meals.

PARSNIP

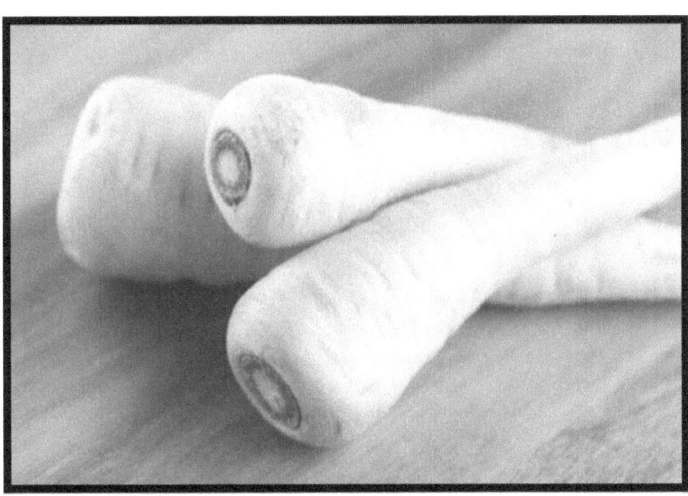

Parsnip is a root vegetable, a member of the umberliferae family, related to carrots, fennel, celeriac, and chervil. Parsnip resembles carrot but is paler and sweeter than carrot and has a nutty flavour.

Parsnip is native to Eurasia, where it has been known for several centuries. Parsnip means forked turnip. It is grown for its sweet, succulent underground taproots.

Parsnip can be eaten raw but is more commonly cooked, boiled, fried, roasted, or added to the soups.

Parsnip is richer in fibre and potassium than carrots. It has less calories, protein, and vitamin C but more fibre and folic acid than potatoes.

Parsnip is a rich source of fibre, vitamins (C, E, K, folic acid, vitamin B6) and minerals (manganese, potassium, copper, magnesium, phosphorus, calcium, iron, selenium).

Parsnip is an excellent source of fibre (16.5 g per serving) and thus it improves digestive tract health, lowers cholesterol, and prevents colon cancer.

Parsnip contains polyacetylene antioxidants that have antifungal, anti-inflammatory and anticancer activity against colon cancer and ALL

Parwal (Green Potato, Pointed Gourd)

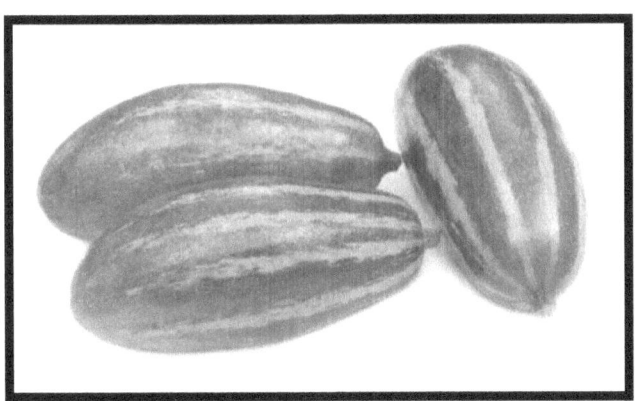

Parwal is a vegetable native to India that resembles cucumber and squash. It has tapering ends, hard green skin, and white or green stripes along its length. It has creamy flesh, heart-shaped leaves, and tiny seeds. The fruit varies in size from five to fifteen centimetres.

Parwal is used as an ingredient in soups, stews, curries, fried dishes, sweets, and stuffing.

Parwal is a rich source of fibre, vitamins (A, C, B1, and B2), and minerals (calcium, magnesium, phosphorus, potassium, iron, copper, and sulphur).

It is low in calories, fat, and cholesterol.

It is a good appetizer.

It enhances digestion.

It relieves constipation.

It stimulates the liver.

It lowers the temperature.

Extracts of parwal seeds improve the levels of blood cholesterol and glucose.

POTATO

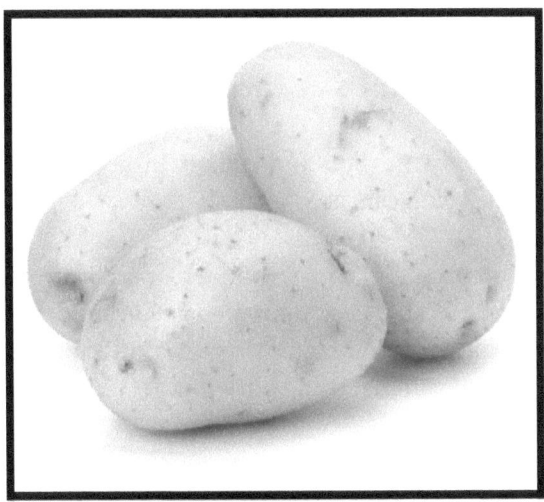

Potato belongs to the nightshade family, which also includes eggplants, tomatoes, and peppers. Potato was cultivated in South America more than 4,000 years ago.

Potato is the swollen portion of a tuber. The tubers have a round, oval, or oblong shape, which vary in size and colour (white, yellow, red). The flesh could also be white or red, having different flavours. There are more than 100 varieties of potatoes available.

Potatoes are a good source of fibre, vitamin C, vitamin B6, manganese, potassium, copper, tryptophan, and flavonoids.

Potatoes are good for health if eaten boiled or baked but are harmful if eaten as French fries or potato chips or eaten with butter, sour cream, or gravy, which add a lot more calories and unhealthy fats. Moreover, French fries may contain a toxic substance, called acrylamide, which is formed in high temperature.

Potatoes contain complex carbohydrates that are filling and provide a moderate amount of energy (twenty-six calories per potato).

Potatoes contain compounds called kukoamines, which lower blood pressure.

The presence of flavonoids, fibre, and vitamin B6 has synergistic effect in lowering the risk of heart attack and stroke.

The fibre in potato aids in digestion, assists in regular bowel movement, and prevents against colon cancer.

Potato is rich in vitamin B6 and tryptophan needed for healthy nervous system and elevated mood. These nutrients are involved in the synthesis of neurotransmitters, such as serotonin (for mood regulation), adrenaline (which responds to stress), and gamma amino butyric acid (GABA) (for relaxation).

Vitamin C and phytochemicals in potato boost immunity and fight infections.

The skin of potato has sixty different phytochemicals and vitamins and should be included in the diet whenever potato is consumed.

PUMPKIN

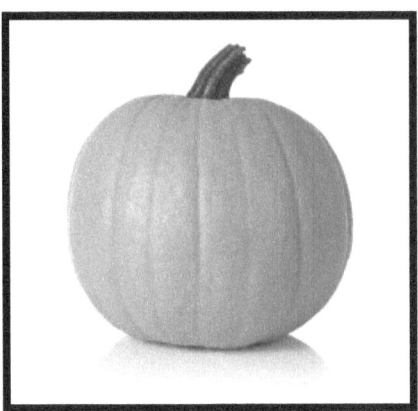

Pumpkin is a fruit that belongs to the gourd family, which also includes squash, cucumber, and melon, but it is used as a vegetable. The word pumpkin is derived from the Greek word *peponi*, meaning a large melon. Pumpkin is native to North America. Pumpkin seeds have been discovered in Mexico dating back to 7,000 years ago.

Pumpkin varies greatly in shape (round, oblong), weight (half a kilogram to twenty-five kilogram), and colour (orange, yellow, green, brown, white, grey, and red).

The rind is thick and smooth with vertical ribs. The fruit has a hollow centre with numerous small whitish seeds, called pepitas.

Pumpkin is cultivated for both consumption and recreation, as in Halloween. Pumpkin can be eaten as a pie, soups, smoothies, muffins, cookies, breads, etc.

Pumpkin is one of the most nutritious fruits available packed with flavonoids (carotene, lutein, zeaxanthin), vitamins (A, C, E, B), minerals (potassium, magnesium, calcium, phosphorus, iron), and fibre.

Beta-cryptoxanthin lowers the risk of lung cancer in smokers. Pumpkin seeds lower the risk of prostate cancer.

Antioxidant contents of pumpkin aid in lowering the severity of arthritis and asthma.

Phytochemicals, potassium, and fibre prevent the onset of cardiovascular diseases and stroke.

Phytochemicals lower blood glucose level and is an aid to diabetics.

Vitamins A and C, manganese, and carotenoids improve the immunity against infections.

Carotenoids help delay the onset of cataract and macular degeneration.

Calcium, magnesium, phosphorus, potassium, zinc, and copper help formation of strong bones and prevention of osteoporosis.

Vitamins A, C, and E and zinc prevent wrinkles and keep skin hydrated and nourished, creating glowing skin.

Pumpkin is a natural diuretic and helps flush out toxins and prevents formation of calcium oxalate stones.

Pumpkin seeds are a good source of proteins, copper, magnesium, and zinc. Pumpkin seed oil is rich in essential fatty acids and tryptophan.

PURSLANE (CAT'S TONGUE)

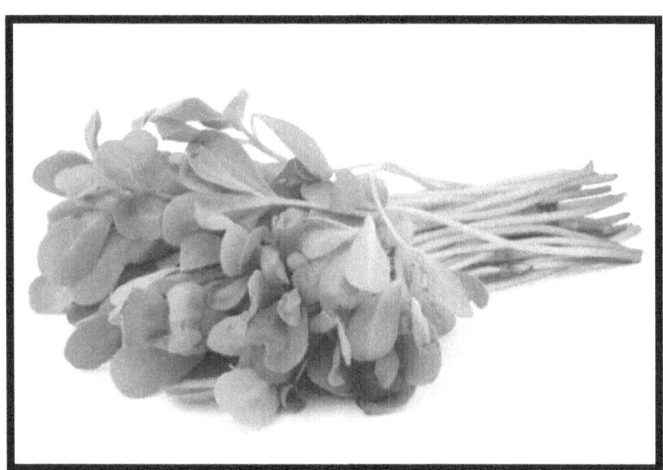

Purslane grows as a weed but is consumed as a vegetable. It is native to India. Purslane has thick, succulent, slightly salty, sour-tasting leaves. The leaves vary in size, thickness, leaf arrangement, and pigment distribution. It has succulent reddish-brown stems and yellow flower buds. Stems, leaves, and buds are all edible.

Purslane has more omega-3 fatty acids than any other leafy vegetable. It is rich in fibre, vitamins (A, C, B), and minerals (iron, magnesium, calcium, potassium, manganese).

Two types of the antioxidant betalain alkaloid pigments are found in purslane, namely, the reddish beta-cyanins and the yellow beta-xanthins that have been found to be antimutagenic.

Purslane has several-fold melatonins than any other vegetable or fruit. Melatonin is a powerful antioxidant that may inhibit tumour growth. Melatonin is a hormone which is also made in the brain and sets the body clock to control sleep cycle.

RADICCHIO

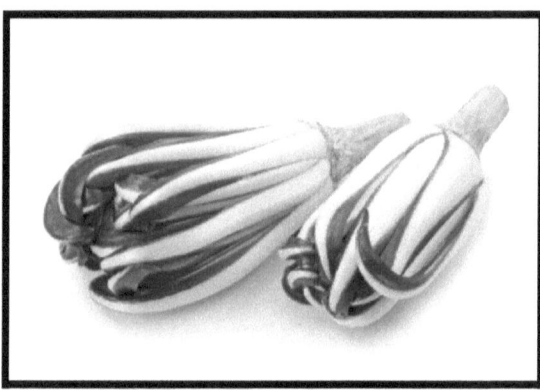

Radicchio is a red leafy vegetable with white veins that belong to the daisy family. It looks like a small red cabbage, about the size of romaine lettuce head. Its leaves are thinner and tenderer than the red cabbage. Red cabbage has reddish purple leaves with a flavour and texture similar to green cabbage, while radicchio has a spicy bitter flavour.

Radicchio originated in Italy, hence referred to as Italian chicory. Some types of chicory plants are cultivated for their leafy vegetables, but some others are grown for their roots, which are baked and ground to be used as a coffee substitute. There are nineteen varieties of radicchio; most of them are named after different regions in Italy.

Radicchio can be eaten raw in salads, sautéed, roasted, or grilled.

It has a unique compound called intybin, which has a sedative analgesic effect and is a potent antimalarial agent.

The anthocyanin content that gives red colour to radicchio is a potent antioxidant.

Radicchio is a rich source of fibre, flavonoids, vitamin K, potassium, copper, and manganese but is low in calories and devoid of fats and cholesterol.

RADISH

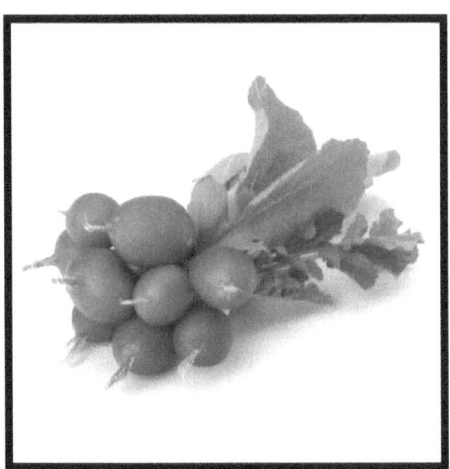

Radish is an edible root vegetable belonging to the cabbage family. The word radish originated from the Latin word *radix*, meaning root. Radish was cultivated in China 3,000 years ago and was given to Japan as a gesture of goodwill.

Radish comes in numerous shapes (round or elongated), sizes, tastes (pungent or sweet), and colours (white, pink, red, purple, black, or green).

Radish can be eaten raw, cooked, juiced, and pickled.

Radish is rich in fibre, vitamins (C and B), minerals (zinc, phosphorus, iron, magnesium, copper, calcium, and potassium), and phytochemicals (anthocyanins, carotenoids, sulphoraphanes, indoles, and isothiocyanates).

Radish has a role in fighting some types of cancers, such as kidney and gastrointestinal tract.

Radish is effective in treating dry skin, rash, cracks, and leucoderma (white skin patches).

Radish contains sulphur compounds, which regulate the production and flow of bile.

Radish can halt the destruction of red blood cells and increase the supply of oxygen to the blood.

Radish helps to relieve congestion within the respiratory tract, making it useful in treating asthma, bronchitis, and sinusitis.

Radish is a natural mouth and breath freshener.

Radish is a great appetiser.

Radish is a natural diuretic, prevents urinary tract infection, and cleans the kidney of toxins.

Radish treats skin itching if applied locally on the skin.

Radish leaves contain more vitamin C, protein, and calcium than the roots.

Red Orach (Mountain Spinach, French Spinach, Garden Orach)

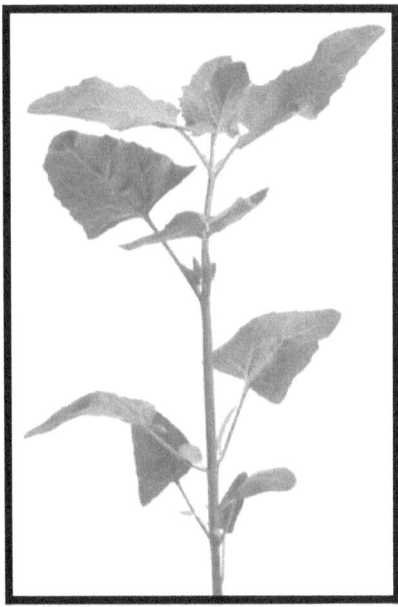

Red orach is a leaf vegetable with a salty, buttery, spinach-like taste, which was originated in Asia and Europe. It is related to lamb's quarters.

The leaves are soft, thick, oblong, triangular, and goosefoot-shaped and are pointed at the ends. The colour is burgundy.

The leaves are used in salads or are baked.

Red orach is rich in fibre, protein, calcium, phosphorus, iron, magnesium, potassium, manganese, copper, zinc, selenium, and vitamins A, C, B, K, and E.

Rhubarb (Pie Plant)

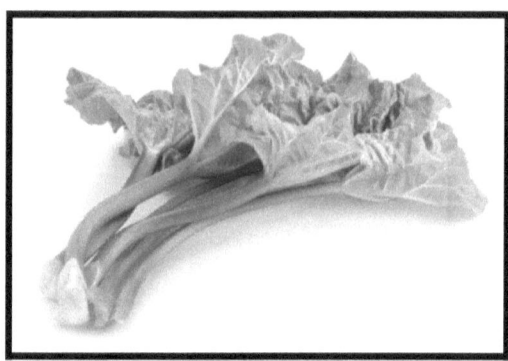

Rhubarb looks like celery but has attractive, succulent rose-red colour and large, heart-shaped leaves. Rhubarb is native to Siberia. It was cultivated more than 4,000 years ago in China for its medicinal values.

The stalks (petioles) are crispy and sour and are used in pies, jams, and jellies.

Rhubarb is rich in fibre, vitamins C and K, calcium, lutein, and lycopene. However, the calcium in rhubarb is not absorbed from the guts because it is combined with oxalic acid.

Anthraquinones in rhubarb have a strong laxative effect. Rhubarb capsule can be used to treat constipation naturally.

Polyphenols in rhubarb have an antileukemia activity. Lycopene in red stalks fights against prostate cancer.

Eating rhubarb lowers blood cholesterol level by inhibiting certain enzymes involved in cholesterol synthesis.

Lutein prevents the damage to eyes by neutralising the free radicals.

Rhubarb can be effective in treating hot flushes in postmenopausal women.

Rhubarb speeds up the metabolism, thus aiding in weight loss.

RUTABAGA (SWEDE, SWEDISH TURNIP, YELLOW TURNIP)

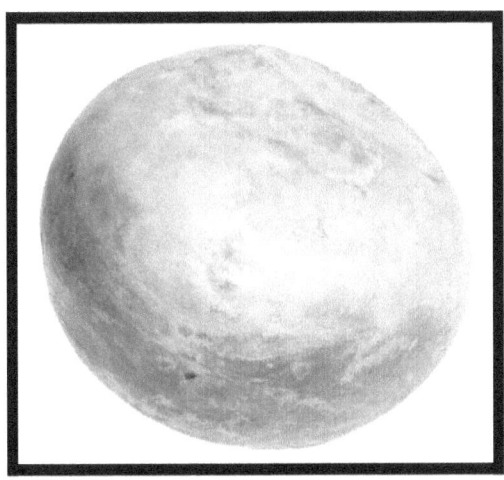

Rutabaga is a root vegetable that belongs to the cabbage family, which was originated as a cross between cabbage and turnip. The name rutabaga has been derived from the Swedish word *rotabagge*, meaning root bag. Rutabaga is native to Russia and Scandinavia.

Rutabaga is closely related to turnips but is larger, rounder, fleshier, and sweeter than turnips and has yellow colour.

Rutabaga can be eaten raw, roasted, stewed, mashed, baked, fried, or added to soups and salads. Even the leaves are edible and nutritious.

Rutabaga is a rich source of fibre, vitamins (C and B), minerals (potassium, phosphorus, manganese, and magnesium), and phytochemicals (carotenoids, isothiocyanates, and glucosinolate).

Rutabaga lowers the risk of colon cancer, type 2 diabetes, heart disease, stroke, constipation, osteoporosis, infections, and Alzheimer's disease.

Rutabaga decreases the frequency of migraine attacks.

Rutabaga increases milk production in nursing mothers.

Rutabaga decreases premenstrual symptoms.

Rutabaga aids in the prevention of spot baldness (alopecia).

SAMPHIRE

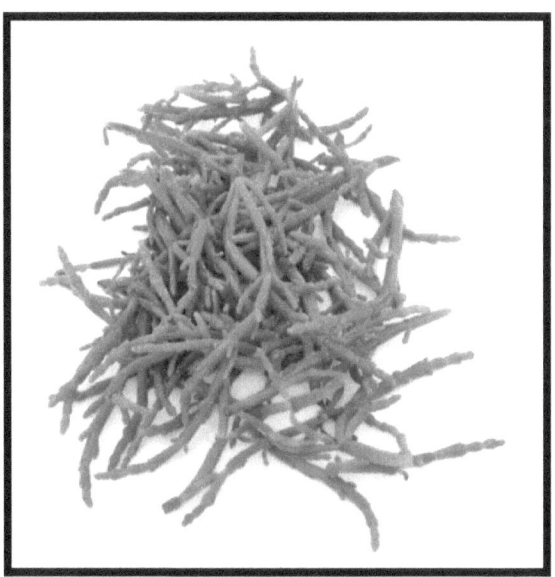

Samphire has succulent, wild, bright-green, shining, aromatic leaflets with tiny yellowish green blossoms, which grow on coastal marshes of Great Britain and on rock cliffs. Samphire looks like a miniature cactus without the spines. It resembles asparagus and hence is called sea asparagus or poor man's asparagus.

In fourteenth century, its ash was used to make glasses; hence, it was called glasswort.

The word 'samphire' was originated from *sampierre*, for the French Saint Pierre, or Saint Peter, the patra saint of fishermen.

March samphire belongs to the same family as beets and chard, while rock samphire belongs to the carrot family.

Samphire has a unique, delicious, salty flavour and crunchy texture. It is used in salads or pickles.

Samphire is a rich source of fibre, vitamins (A, C, and some B), minerals (iron, calcium, magnesium, iodine, phosphorus, zinc, silicon, and Manganese), amino acids, linoleic acid, quercetin, isorhamnetin, and glycosides.

Phytochemicals protect liver, heart, and DNA.

Glycosides have anticancer properties.

It aids in digestion and relieves flatulence (carminative) like fennel.

It is a natural diuretic.

It boosts energy.

It is a blood purifier and cleanser (depurative).

Scallions (Green Onions, Spring Onions)

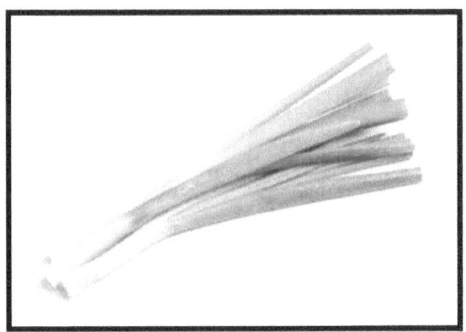

Scallions belong to the allium family, which includes onion, shallot, garlic, and chive. Scallions are young, immature onions with a small white tip harvested very early before the plant forms a large bulb. Scallions have long, slender, hollow, tubular green stalks that look like giant chives.

Scallions have milder flavour than onions but stronger than chives.

Scallions are a good source of vitamins (A, C, K, and folic acid), minerals (calcium, iron, copper, and manganese), carotenoids, and some omega-3 fatty acids.

They lower the risk of gastrointestinal tract cancer.

They are cardioprotective.

They aid in normal blood clot formation.

They are anti-allergic.

They aid in DNA synthesis.

They are a good appetiser.

SEA BEET

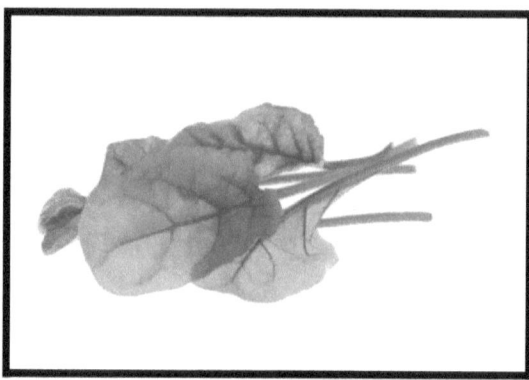

Sea beet is the wild ancestor of beetroot, sugar beet, and Swiss chard. Sea beet has triangular or oval, glossy leaves, green flowers, and reddish stems.

Sea beet is native to the coast of Europe, Northern Africa, and southern India.

Sea beet has a pleasant texture and flavour whether eaten raw or cooked. All parts of sea beet can be eaten, including roots and flowers.

Sea beet is a rich source of fibre, vitamins (A, C, K, and folic acid), and minerals (iron, copper, magnesium, and potassium).

SEA VEGETABLES

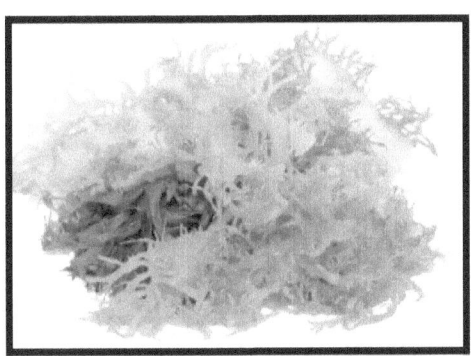

Sea vegetables are the miraculous sea weeds that grow in or near the sea and in some fresh water lakes. They have been eaten for food for thousands of years. Sea vegetables are a type of algae that are harvested, dried, and processed for human consumption in salads, soups, stews, and stir-fries. They are even found in processed forms as thickeners and stabilisers in ice cream, puddings, whipped toppings, salad dressings, and toothpastes.

Sea vegetables have been an ingredient in Japanese dishes for over 10,000 years. Since Japan is the largest producer and exporter of sea vegetables, they mostly have Japanese names.

There are thousands of types of sea vegetables with different shape, taste, texture, and colour (brown, red, green, blue-green, purple, and black).

Sea vegetables are superior in nutrient content than land vegetables and contain elements that are often lacking in land vegetables due to soil depletion. People living in areas where sea vegetables are regularly consumed tend to live longer and healthier lives.

Sea vegetables are low in calories and have no fat but are rich sources of protein, fibre, vitamins (K, A, C, and B), minerals (iron, calcium, and magnesium), trace elements (iodine, silicon, zinc, manganese, copper, and selenium), fucans, alginates, lignans, and ergosterol.

Some of the most popular sea vegetables are as follows:

Alaria (Winged Kelp)

Alaria is a brown algae dried and used as a food in Western Europe, China, Korea, Japan, and South America.

Arame

Arame is a dark brown lacy alga with a sweet flavour and firm texture.

Bladderwrack

Bladderwrack is a brown seaweed similar to kelp. It is one of the most common algae on the shores of the British Isles. It gets its name from the air sacs that keep the plants afloat in cold sea water. It is used in steam baths to decrease arthritic pain.

Dulse

Dulse is a red salty alga that grows in the Northern Atlantic and the coasts of the Pacific Ocean.

Hijiki

Hijiki is a brown cylindrical alga that resembles hair. It has a firm texture and intense aroma. It has the highest concentration of calcium of all sea vegetables. It has high levels of contaminated heavy metals and cannot be eaten raw.

Irish Moss (Carrageen Moss)

It is a red alga that grows in Europe and North America.

Kelp

Kelp is a large, tree-like, brown alga that grows in shallow ocean on the Pacific coasts.

Kombu (King of Sea Weeds)

Kombu is a dark green, long, thick alga from the kelp family. It is a Japanese delicacy, an essential ingredient of dashi, a flavourful stock, which forms the base for miso soup, clear broth, and noodle broth. Kombu is rich in glutamic acid, the basis of monosodium glutamate (MSG), which is widely used in processed foods.

Laver

Laver is a purple seaweed that is harvested in the British Isles. It is unusual because the leaves are only one cell thick. Laver is closely related to nori, used as sushi wrapper in Japan.

Nori

Nori is a red alga that is the mildest form of seaweeds with a sweet meaty flavour. It has the highest content of proteins (50%) in sea plants. Nori is used in Japan for wrapping sushi.

Sea Palm (Postelsia)

Sea palm is a large brown kelp that grows on rocking shores along the western coast of North America. It is one of the few algae that can survive outside the water.

Wakame

Wakame is a thin stringy alga, is deep green in colour, and has a subtly sweet taste, which is used in salads and soups. Wakame is used in the Orient for hair lustre and growth and skin tone.

Sea vegetables share the following properties:

- They are fat-free and have low calorie, great for losing weight.
- They have high content of complete protein with all the essential amino acids, similar to meat protein.

- They have high iodine content for maintaining thyroid health.
- Alginic acid binds to heavy metals and radionucleotides and flushes them outside the body, thus preventing them from damaging DNA.
- Lignans bind to oestrogen receptors in the breast, thus lowering the oestrogen's ability to stimulate breast tissue to form tumour. Additionally, fucoidan interferes with the ability of cells to proliferate.
- Fucoidans are sulphated polysaccharides that have anti-inflammatory, anticoagulant, and antithrombotic properties, which keep cardiovascular health.
- Ergosterol from sea vegetables converts in the body to vitamin D.
- Sea vegetables strengthen hair, nail, and skin.
- They are great liver detoxifiers.
- They boost sex drive.
- Hazards of eating large quantities of sea vegetables include goitre enlargement by excessive intake of iodine, increasing blood pressure, and heart failure by high sodium intake, and ingestion of heavy metal contaminants, including arsenic, cadmium, mercury, and lead.

SHALLOTS (MADRAS ONIONS)

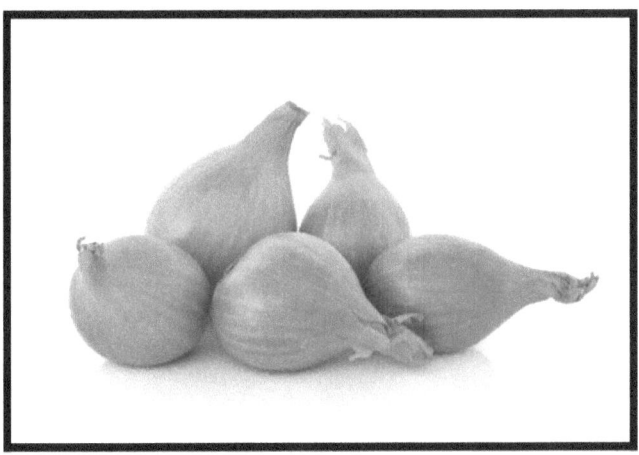

Shallots are long, slender bulbs in the allium family of root vegetables, which also includes onions, garlic, chives, and scallions. They are miniature forms of onions. They grow in clusters of bulbs attached at the base by loose skins. After peeling, shallots divide into two to six cloves like garlic, rather than onion.

The skin colour of shallots varies from golden brown to grey to rose red.

Shallots are less pungent than onion or garlic. The flavour is actually a combination of sweet onion and garlic.

Shallots originated in the Mediterranean region and Central Asia.

Shallots are used in cooking, pickled, or deep-fried.

Shallots have more antioxidants, vitamins, and minerals than onions. They are a rich source of flavonoid antioxidants (quercetin and kaempferol) and sulphur compounds that convert to allicin in the body.

Soybean (Soya Bean)
(The King of Beans)

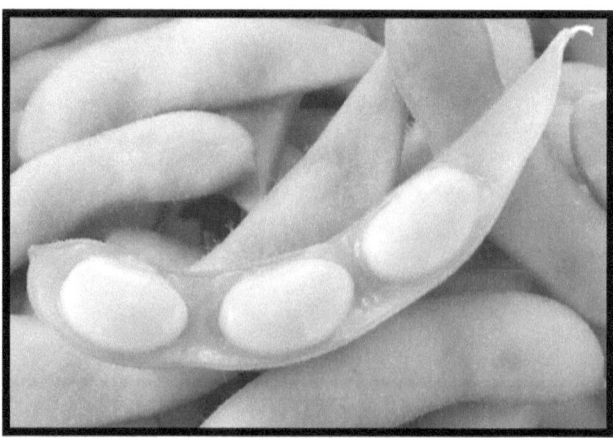

Soybean is a legume of the pea family that originated in China thousands of years ago. There are two to four beans per pod. Soybean comes in many sizes and colours (green, brown, black, blue, yellow, and mottled).

Fermentation techniques were discovered in China to increase digestibility of soybeans by making soy sauce, soy paste, natto, tempeh, miso and tamari. Non-fermented products, like soy milk and tofu, are also available. Besides, soybean is used in many foods, like soy hotdogs, soy burgers, soy cheese, soy yogurt and soy ice cream or processed to make soy oil, soy flour and soy meal.

Soybeans are a good source of fibre (42%), Protein (36%), oil (19%), omega-3 fatty acids, vitamins (K, C and B2), minerals (calcium, magnesium, phosphorus, potassium, molybdenum, manganese, and copper), isoflavones (genistein, dainzein, and glycitein), phytosterols, saponins, and lecithin.

Soybean is regarded as the 'plant meat'. It has higher protein content than other legumes and is the only plant source of complete protein. Soybean has 36% protein, soy flour has 40 to 50% protein, soy protein has 70% protein, and soy protein isolate has 90% protein.

Isoflavones lower the risk of breast, ovarian, and prostate cancers. Sphingolipids and fibre lower the risk of colon cancer. Protease inhibin inhibits several forms of cancer. Saponins are antioxidants that inhibit the growth of tumour cells.

Glycitein is a phytoestrogen that has a weak oestrogenic activity that can ease the postmenopausal symptoms, such as hot flashes, osteoporosis, and heart diseases in women.

Omega-3 fatty acids, lecithin, phytoestrogens, fibre, and potassium work synergistically to lower the risk of heart diseases.

Isoflavones slow down skin ageing, and linoleic acid prevents melanin synthesis in the skin.

Lecithin is an important component of brain cells, thus having a role in preventing Alzheimer's disease. Phytosterols increase the function of nerve cells.

Lecithin promotes absorption of fat-soluble vitamins from the gut.

SPINACH

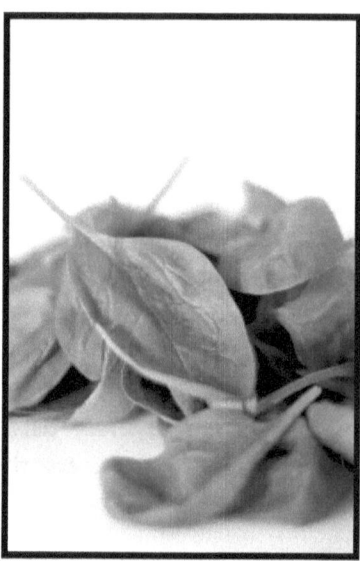

Spinach belongs to the goosefoot family, which also includes Swiss chard and beet greens, and tastes like them. Spinach originated in ancient Persia. It has dark green tender leaves, which can be eaten raw when young.

Spinach is a rich source of protein (the highest vegetable source of protein (5 g per cup), fibre (20% of RDA), vitamin K (second only to cauliflower, providing 1000% of RDA), vitamin A, vitamin C, minerals (manganese, magnesium, iron, calcium, phosphorus, copper, and zinc), carotenoids (lutein, neoxanthin, and beta-carotene), flavonoids (such as kaempferol), and omega-3 fatty acids.

Glycoglycerolipids have special protective effect against inflammation and cancer of gastrointestinal tract. Kaempferol lowers the risk of ovarian cancer. Fibre and vitamins A and C protect against colon cancer. Flavonoids also slow down cell division in stomach and skin, thus preventing carcinoma of these organs.

Spinach contains powerful antioxidants, such as vitamin A, vitamin C, manganese, and zinc, which protect the body against free radical damage.

Neoxanthin, vialaxanthin, and omega-3 fatty acids regulate inflammatory processes in the body.

Due to the presence of some peptides in spinach, blood pressure is lowered.

Flavones in spinach prevent harmful effect of oxidation on the brain, protecting it from premature ageing.

Some benefits of spinach are as follows:

+ Healthy vision
+ Immunity boosting
+ Healthy bones
+ Healthy nervous system
+ Healthy skin
+ Healthy heart
+ Correction of anaemia
+ Constipation prevention

SQUASH

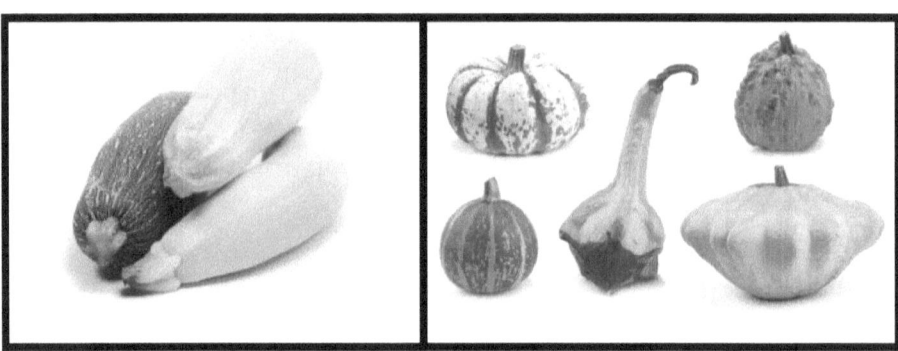

Squash belongs to the gourd family, which includes pumpkin, cucumber, and melon. Squash is actually a fruit, but it is used as vegetable. Squash is indigenous to Mexico. Its seeds have been recovered from Mexican caves dating back to more than 10,000 years.

Squash are of two types: summer squash and winter squash. Both of them come in a variety of colours and sizes. The varieties of summer squash include zucchini, crookneck, straight neck, and patty pan. Winter squash varieties include butternut, acorn, hubbard, turban, and spaghetti. Summer squash has a thin edible skin, soft seeds, and high water content. Winter squash has a thick rind, giving it a long storage life, which could extend for months. Winter squash is sweeter and more nutritious (having more beta-carotene and B vitamins) than summer squash.

Squash is a good source of fibre, vitamins (C, A, B), minerals (potassium, magnesium, phosphorus, manganese, zinc, copper, iron, calcium), omega-3 fatty acids, tryptophan, protein, lutein, and zeaxanthin. Summer squash should be eaten with seeds and the skin to derive maximum health benefits.

Beta-cryptoxanthin lowers the risk of lung cancer.

Squash lowers the symptoms of enlarged prostate.

Carotenoids lower the risk of cataract and macular degeneration.

B vitamins, fibre, zinc, magnesium, and omega-3 fatty acids all assist in controlling blood glucose level in type 2 diabetes.

Vitamins A, C, B6, and B9, fibre, magnesium, and potassium protect heart from heart attack.

Calcium, phosphorus, magnesium, copper, manganese, and zinc aid in healthy bone formation and energy production.

B vitamins act as cofactors in the metabolism of carbohydrates, protein, and fat, hence energy production.

It is an immunity booster.

Tryptophan in squash helps mental relaxation and sleep.

Sweet Potato

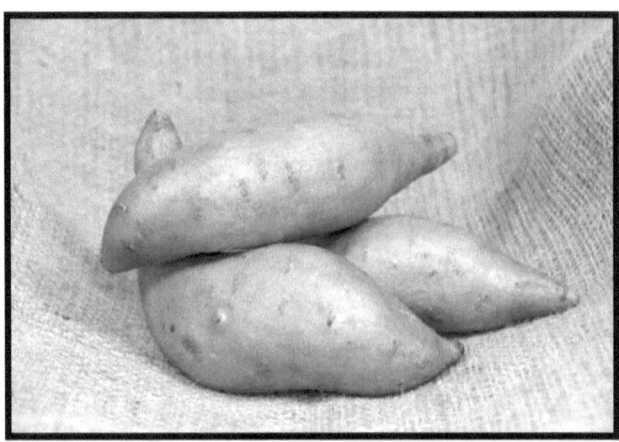

Sweet potato is native to Central America and has a history of more than 5,000 years. It is the world's sixth largest food crop and is important for the growing population in Asian and African countries.

Despite its name, sweet potato is not related to potato. While potato is a tuber, sweet potato is a root.

Sweet potato has an oblong, elongated shape with tapering ends and a smooth skin, whose colour ranges from yellow, orange, red, brown to purple. The flesh can be white, yellow, orange, pink, red, purple, or violet.

Sweet potato can be eaten boiled, grilled, fried, roasted, and baked.

Sweet potato is a rich source of fibre, vitamins (C, A, and B6), minerals (manganese, potassium, calcium, iron, magnesium, and copper), beta-carotene, and polyphenols like anthocyanins and phenolic acid.

Although sweet, it can regulate blood glucose level.

It fights colon, intestine, kidney, and prostate cancers.

It boosts immunity.

It relieves asthma.

It relieves arthritic pain to certain extent.

It maintains healthy skin.

It prevents vision problems.

It prevents constipation.

It prevents heart disease.

It prevents stomach ulcer.

The leaves of sweet potato are also edible and are more nutritious than some of the green leafy vegetables.

SWISS CHARD (SILVERBEET)

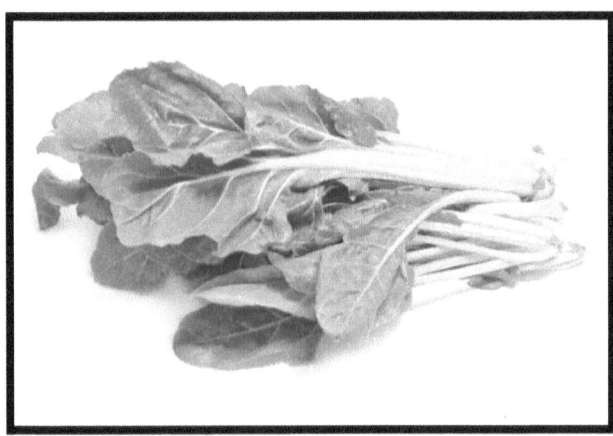

Swiss chard, or simply chard, is a member of the goosefoot family and is a relative of beets and spinach. Chard has fleshy, tender, deep green leaves and thick, crispy edible stalks, which come in many colours, including white, green, yellow, orange, pink, red, purple, or rainbow.

Chard is native to Sicily and not Switzerland. It was called Swiss chard by the Swiss botanist in honour of his country.

Chard is rich in fibre, vitamins (K, A and C), minerals (magnesium, potassium, iron, calcium, phosphorus, manganese, and boron), carotenoids (carotenes, lutein, zeaxanthin, and quercetin), omega-3 fatty acids, and syringic acid.

Chard prevents colon and prostate cancers.

It prevents heart diseases.

It prevents type 2 diabetes.

It prevents vision disorders.

It prevents Alzheimer's disease.

It prevents weight gain.

It prevents anaemia.

It prevents osteoporosis.

It prevents infections.

It prevents alopecia (hair loss).

Taro (Elephant Ears)

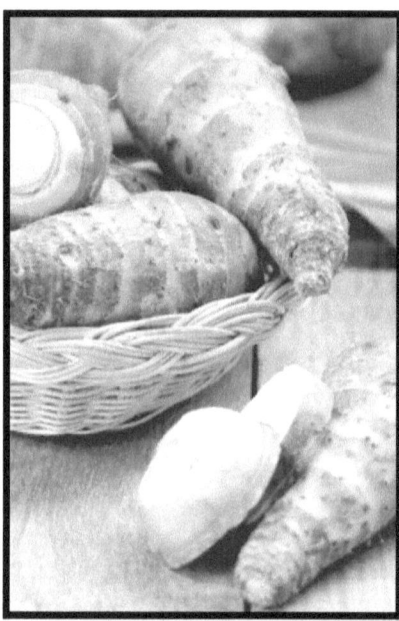

Taro is native to South-East Asia and is considered a staple food in Africa, Asia, and Pacific Islands for 10% of world's population.

Taro is a starchy, globular or oblong, fleshy, underground root of the aroid family.

Taro is grown for its delicious, crunchy, nutty tuber or corm, which tastes like water chestnut. The corm grows to the size of turnip, weighing as much as one kilogram.

Taro has a brown fibrous skin and a white to creamy yellow flesh.

Taro corms and leaves must be boiled before consumption to leach out the toxic calcium oxalate crystals, which could precipitate kidney stones.

Taro is considered as the potato humid tropics. Taro corms are roasted, boiled, baked, or made into cakes and chips.

Taro has more fibre and calories than potato but has lower glycemic index, making it better than potato for diabetic patients. The calories in taro come from amylase and amylopectin.

Taro is low in fats and protein but rich in vitamins (C, E, and B), minerals (calcium, magnesium, manganese, copper, phosphorus, iron, zinc, and selenium), and omega-3 fatty acids.

Taro leaves contain fibre, vitamins A and C, protein, beta-carotene, and cryptoxanthin.

Tinda (Indian Round Gourd, Indian Baby Pumpkin, Indian Apple Gourd)

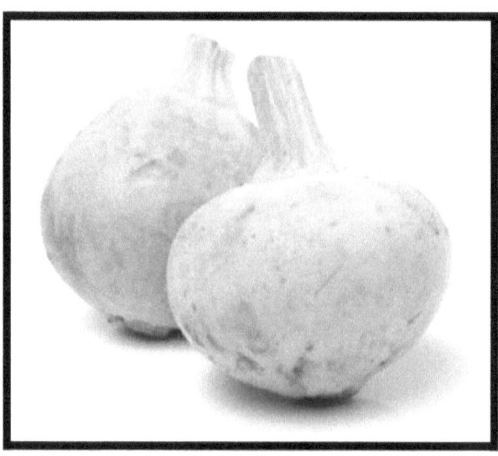

Tinda is a squash-like gourd, popular in India and Pakistan, grown for its immature fruit. It is light green, apple-sized, flattish round. The skin is tough, and the flesh is firm and snow white in colour. It has a tasty nutty flavour.

Tinda can be stewed, pickled, stuffed, juiced, or candied. The seeds may also be roasted and eaten.

Tinda is rich in fibre, antioxidants, and anti-inflammatory compounds.

Tinda lowers the risk of heart disease, stroke, and some types of cancers. It also aids in controlling blood pressure.

TOMATO

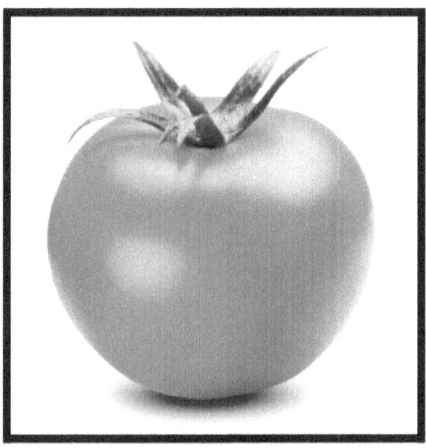

Tomato originated in South America, but China is now the producer of tomato. Botanically, tomato is a berry fruit, but it is consumed as a vegetable. Tomato belongs to the nightshade family, which also includes potato, eggplant, and peppers. There are more than 7,500 varieties of tomatoes based on their shape, size, and colour. Although tomato is usually red, it can be yellow, orange, or green. Some of the varieties of tomatoes include globe, beefsteak, oxheart, roma, campari, pear-shaped, plum-shaped, cherry-shaped, and grape-shaped.

Tomato can be eaten raw, canned, juiced, sauced, and added to soups.

Tomato is a good source of fibre, tryptophan, protein, vitamins (C, A, K, folic acid, and E), minerals (potassium, molybdenum, manganese, copper, magnesium, phosphorus, and iron), carotenoids (lycopene, beta-carotene, lutein, and zeaxanthin), and other phytochemicals. Lycopene, which imparts the red colour to tomato, is the highest in tomato than in all the fruits and vegetables.

The absorption of carotenoids and flavonoids from tomato increases after cooking because cooking breaks down the tomato cell matrix and makes these nutrients more available. The addition of oil, such as olive oil, to tomato during cooking increases the absorption of fat-soluble carotenoids.

Lycopene in tomato is a powerful antioxidant, highly effective in scavenging cancer-causing free radicals, especially in fighting prostate, breast, cervix, bladder, and gastrointestinal cancers.

Lycopene lowers the level of cholesterol and triglyceride, thus preventing deposition of fats in blood vessels that could lead to heart attack and stroke.

Certain compounds in tomato fight against nitrosamines, which are the main carcinogens found in cigarette smoke.

It helps healthy vision.

It aids healthy skin.

It aids healthy gut.

It protects from infection.

It controls bleeding by forming normal blood clots.

It helps formation of red blood cells.

It helps in building strong bones.

It is a blood purifier.

It lowers the oxidative stress in type 2 diabetes.

TURNIP

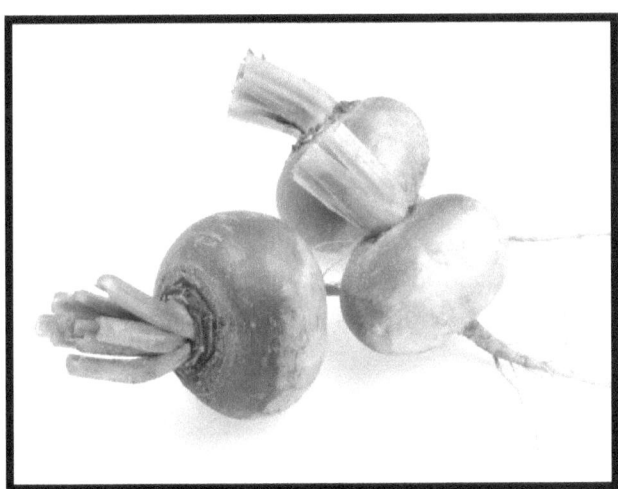

Turnip is a root vegetable belonging to the cruciferae family, which also includes cabbage, kale, Brussels sprout, collards, etc. Turnip is native to Western Asia. It has been used as a food for humans and their livestock for 4,000 years.

Turnip had been a daily staple in Europe before potatoes.

Turnip comes in a variety of shapes (conical or global), sizes (up to one kilogram), and colours (white, purple, pink, or green). If it is yellow, it could be rutabaga.

Turnip resembles potato in texture and appearance but has a bitter flavour with only one-third of the calories of potato.

Turnip is high in fibre, vitamins (C and B), minerals (calcium, iron, manganese, copper, and magnesium), and phytochemicals. Turnip juice has twice as much vitamin C as orange juice.

Antioxidants and phytochemicals lower the risk of some types of cancers, such as stomach, colon, bladder, and lung cancers.

High folic acid and fibre have a beneficial effect on heart health.

Glucosinolates help the stomach prevent the bacterium H. pylori, which causes stomach ulcer.

It aids in forming strong bones.

Turnip greens are much richer than the roots in nutrient content of vitamins (A, K, C, and folic acid), minerals (calcium, copper, iron, and manganese), carotenes, xanthin, lutein, and glucosinolates.

ULLUCO

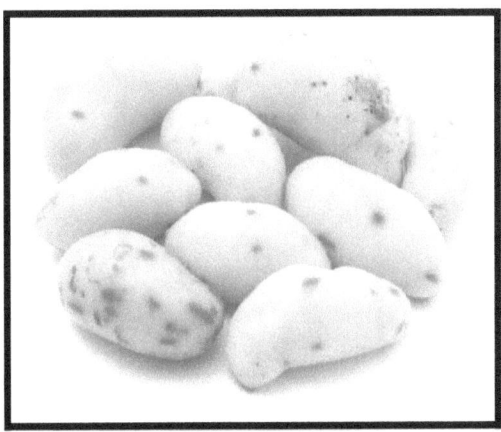

Ulluco is a tuber that is popular in South America for its delicious nutty taste. It is an ingredient in stews and pickles.

The tubers come in a variety of shapes (oblong and round) and colours (white, yellow, brown, red, and green).

The skin is soft and shiny and needs no peeling before eating.

The leaves are green and similar to spinach in texture.

Ulluco is a good source of fibre, protein, calcium, starch, and carotenes.

It helps maintain healthy population of bacteria in the gut.

It lowers the risk of some types of cancers.

It lowers blood cholesterol.

It is an immune booster.

It is a libido enhancer.

Wasabi (Japanese Horseradish)

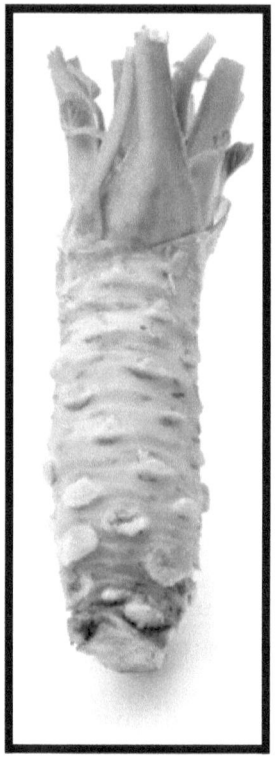

Wasabi is a root vegetable that belongs to the cabbage family. It is native to Japan, where it grows down the length of streambeds in river valleys.

Wasabi is used as a staple condiment and thickening agent in Japan in many traditional dishes like sushi.

Wasabi is a variety of green horseradish grown mostly for its roots. The root is ground into a paste and served as a paste in sushi restaurants. Its flavour is unique and is used to enhance dips, meats, and other foods. The flavour is hotter, and the smell is stronger than the common white horseradish and burns the nose.

The leaves are serrated and have brilliant green colour and are used in salad or pickles.

Wasabi is a rich source of fibre, vitamin C, some B vitamins, potassium, calcium, phosphorus, beta-carotene, isothiocyanates, and glucosinolates.

Isothiocyanates and glucosinolates lower the risk of breast and prostate cancers.

Wasabi stops the growth of bacteria that cause food poisoning and dental caries.

Wasabi prevents abnormal blood clot formation and thus lowers the risk of developing heart attack and stroke.

Wasabi has anti-inflammatory properties and lowers the symptoms of arthritis, asthma, and allergic reactions.

Wasabi has a mucolytic action and thus lowers mucous in airway passages.

Wasabi treats congested sinuses.

Wasabi is an appetiser and aids in digestion.

Wasabi relieves constipation.

Wasabi is a diuretic and relieves body of toxic substances.

WATER CHESTNUT

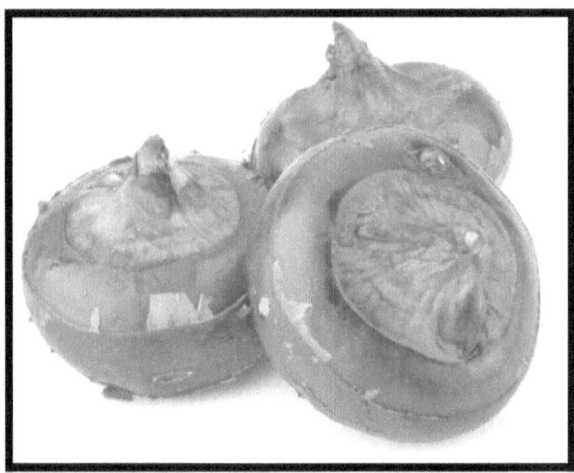

Water chestnut is a tuber vegetable that resembles chestnut in shape and colour. It is an aquatic plant grown for it roots (corms) in fresh water ponds, marshes, lakes, and streams.

Water chestnut originated in South-East Asia. It is a popular ingredient in Chinese dishes.

This knobby vegetable has a papery brown skin. The small round corms have a crisp, crunchy, white, slightly sweet flesh, which can be eaten raw, grilled, boiled, pickled, or added to salads, soups, and stuffing.

The corms are rich in carbohydrates (90% of dry weight, mostly starch), protein (3.4%), fibre (15%), vitamin B, potassium, copper, and manganese.

Because of its high carbohydrate content, it is a good source of energy. It is gluten-free, cholesterol-free, and almost fat-free.

WATERCRESS

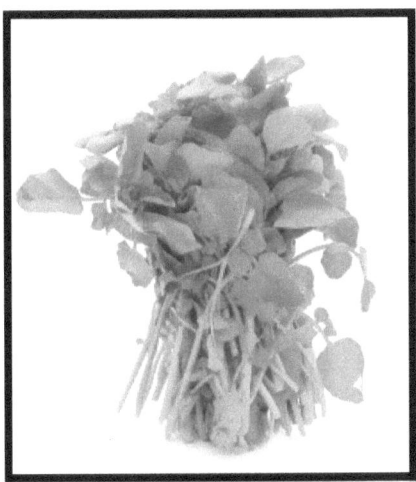

Watercress is a member of the brassica family. Watercress is related to garden cress, mustard, and radish. It resembles broccoli, cabbage, and Brussels sprouts in health benefits.

Watercress is an aquatic vegetable with small, oval, deep-green succulent leaves. The taste is peppery and slightly sour, like mustard greens and garden cress.

Watercress is native to Europe and Asia.

Watercress is usually eaten raw but can also be cooked.

Watercress is rich in vitamins (C, K, and A), minerals (calcium, potassium, magnesium, manganese, and phosphorus), carotenoids (carotenes, lutein, and zeaxanthin), and glucosinolates (the precursors of isothiocyanates).

Watercress is low in calories (11 calories per 100 grams).

Watercress contains a unique phytochemical, nasturtin, which is converted in the body to phenylethyl isothicyanate (PEITC), which inhibits growth of prostate, breast, and colon cancers.

It is an expectorant.

It is a diuretic.

It is a digestive.

WATER SPINACH
(Kangkong, Swamp Cabbage)

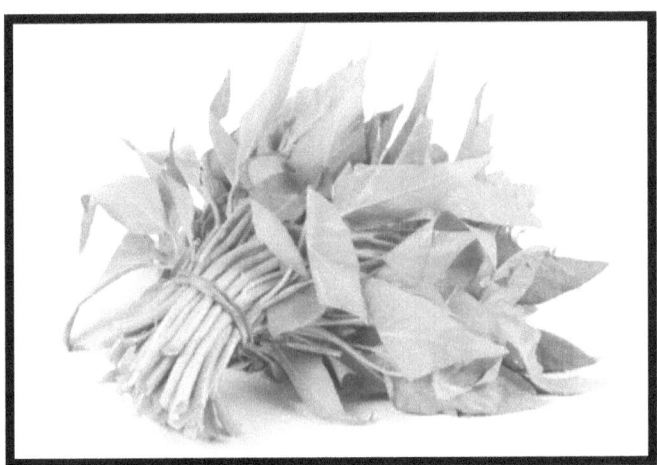

Water spinach is not related to spinach but is closely related to sweet potato. It is a member of the morning glory family. It originated in East India. It is an aquatic or semi-aquatic plant of the tropics and subtropics. It grows easily in marshes, rivers, and streams. In parts of USA, it is considered a noxious weed.

Water spinach has long, jointed, hollow green or white stems, which allow vines to float on water or creep across muddy ground. Its leaves are flat and vary in shape, depending on the variety, from heart-shaped to long, narrow arrow-shaped. It has large attractive white or pink flowers. The leaves have pleasant, mild sweet flavour and slippery texture.

Water spinach is eaten raw or stir-fried.

Water spinach is a rich source of fibre, vitamins (A, C, and B1), iron, calcium, phosphorus, amino acids, sitosterol and carotenoids (carotenes, lutein, violaxanthin, and neoxanthin).

Benefits of water spinach include the following:

- Anticancer
- Antioxidant
- Anti-inflammatory
- Anti-infective
- Antihelmintic (expelling worms from the body)
- Anti-diabetic (because of insulin-like effect)
- Hemostatic (preventing bleeding)
- Laxative
- Diuretic
- Sedative (sleeping effect)
- Decrease in menstrual pain
- Vision health

WHEATGRASS

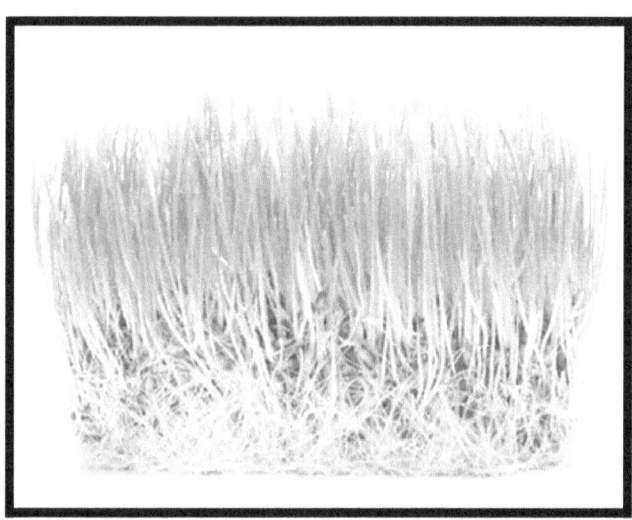

Wheatgrass is a young grass of the common wheat plant. The young wheat seed sprouts of one to weeks old are harvested before stalks form a head with grains. Wheatgrass is consumed as a dried powder or juice. The juice has medicinal value than the powder form because heat destroys the valuable enzymes.

Wheatgrass is rich in vitamins (A, C, and E), minerals (iron, calcium, and magnesium), amino acids, enzymes, and chlorophyll, which constitutes 70% of its weight.

Wheatgrass has a chemical that kills infective agents associated with the common cold, bronchitis, and diarrhoea.

Enzymes in the raw wheatgrass juice neutralise the toxins and carcinogens in the body.

Drinking wheatgrass juice helps in treating infections of the bladder, urethra, kidney, and prostate.

Wheatgrass juice can lower the symptoms of ulcerative colitis, including rectal bleeding. This could be the result of anti-inflammatory action of its antioxidants.

High chlorophyll content stimulates production of red blood cells.

YACON
(The Apple of the Earth)

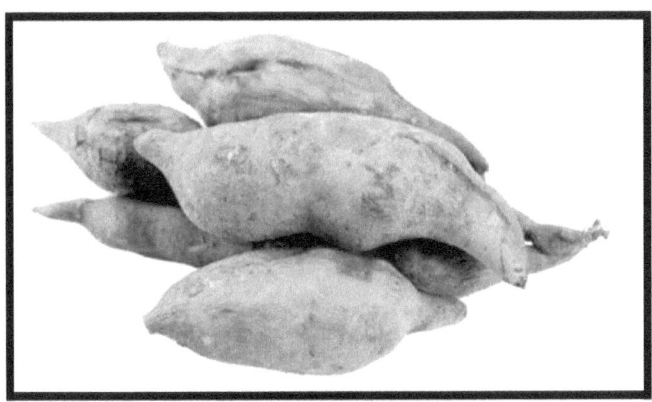

Yacon is a sweet crunchy root vegetable native to South America, particularly Peru. It resembles yam and tastes like a cross between apple and celery. In Peru, it is eaten as a fruit. It can be eaten in fruit salads, stir-fried, roasted, baked, or used in pies and chips.

Yacon tubers can have white, yellow, orange, pink, red, or purple flesh, with distinct flavours.

The huge leaves of yacon are used to wrap foods during cooking, similar to grape leaves used in the Middle East, banana leaves in tropics, and cabbage leaves in Germany.

Yacon is a rich source of fibre, antioxidant vitamins (A, C, and E), and inulin (fructo-oligosaccharides).

Sweet tuberous root is ideal for diabetics and weight watchers due to the presence of inulin that cannot be digested by the body.

Yacon syrup and powder are used as low-calorie sweeteners.

Antioxidant vitamins and chlorogenic and ferulic acids fight the free radicals, which cause oxidation of the cells.

It is an immune booster.

It aids in heart health.

It is antimicrobial.

It is a diuretic.

It protects the liver.

It aids in bone formation.

Yacon leaves lower artery-clogging plaque.

Tea made from the leaves can lower blood glucose by increasing the quantity of insulin circulating in the blood stream.

YAM

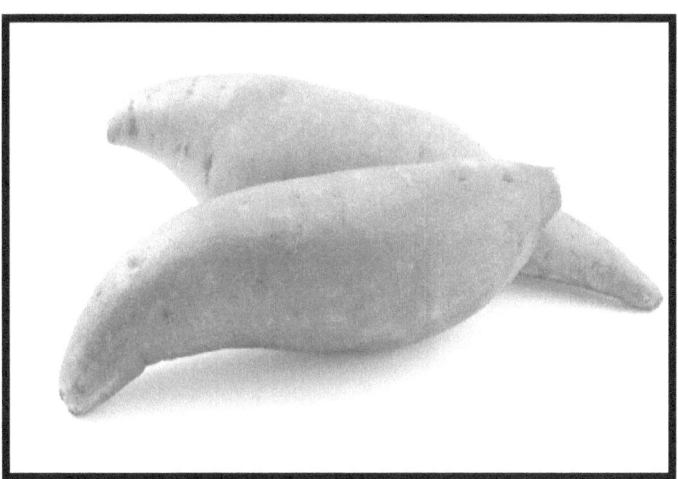

Yam is a staple starchy tuber vegetable native to Africa, Asia, and tropical America.

Yam is similar to sweet potato in appearance but is not related to it at all. Sweet potato is smaller than yam and has a thinner skin, which is edible. The size of yam varies from the size of a small potato to a giant size of fifty kilograms. There are more than 600 varieties of yams, the majority of which is grown in Africa. Nigeria is the largest producer and exporter of yam.

Yam is a rich source of fibre, calories, vitamin C, vitamin B6, potassium, and manganese.

Fibre lowers LDL by binding to it in the intestine, prevents constipation, and decreases the risk of colon cancer.

Yam contains 40 grams of carbohydrates and 263 calories per serving, making it a great source of energy.

The antioxidant vitamin C has an important role in immunity, anti-ageing, wound healing, and bone growth.

Vitamin B6 breaks down homocysteine, the amino acid that could damage blood cell walls, thus lowering the risk of heart attack and stroke.

Potassium is an important component of body fluids that control heart rate and lower blood pressure by counteracting the effects of sodium.

Manganese is a cofactor in a number of enzymatic reactions involved in energy production and antioxidant defences.

Top Twenty Healthy Vegetables

+ Asparagus
+ Bell pepper
+ Broccoli
+ Brussels sprouts
+ Cabbage
+ Carrot
+ Cauliflower
+ Celery
+ Chard
+ Eggplant
+ Garlic
+ Greens (collard greens, mustard greens, turnip greens, and beet greens)
+ Kale
+ Legumes (beans, peas, and lentils)
+ Okra
+ Onion
+ Parsley
+ Spinach
+ Squash
+ Tomato

Vegetable Sources of Nutrients

Vitamin A: carrot, bell pepper, pumpkin, parsley, corn, eggplant, endive, sweet potato, squash, asparagus, green beans and peas, green leafy vegetables, tomato, cucumber.

Vitamin B1: garlic, onion, lettuce, asparagus, mushroom, spinach, tomato, eggplant, Brussels sprout, celery, cabbage, bell pepper, carrot, squash, corn, broccoli, kale.

Vitamin B2: mushroom, squash, lettuce, asparagus, chard, broccoli, collard greens, celery, kale, cabbage, tomato, cauliflower, Brussels sprouts, green beans, and peas.

Vitamin B3: mushroom, asparagus, tomato, squash, green peas, collard greens, carrots, broccoli, spinach, eggplant, cauliflower, kale.

Vitamin B5: corn, mushroom, broccoli, tomato, squash, collard greens, chard.

Vitamin B6: spinach, bell peppers, garlic, cauliflower, broccoli, celery, asparagus, cabbage, mushroom, kale, collard greens, Brussels sprouts, chard, carrot, tomato, squash, eggplant, lettuce.

Vitamin B9: lettuce, spinach, asparagus, collard greens, broccoli, cauliflower, artichoke, beets, celery, legumes, cabbage, bell pepper, tomato.

Vitamin B12: Vegetables do not contain vitamin B12.

Vitamin C: green leafy vegetables, bell peppers, cucumber, tomato, squash, celery, endive, arugula, fennel, dandelion greens, corn, green beans, and peas

Vitamin D: bok choy, mushroom, sea vegetables.

Vitamin E: asparagus, corn, tomato, parsnip, endive, dandelion greens, mustard greens.

Vitamin K: sweet potato, tomato, green leafy vegetables, sea vegetables, legumes, squash, parsley, bell peppers, celery.

Boron: chard.

Calcium: most vegetables.

Chromium: onion, tomato, lettuce, asparagus, bamboo shoots.

Copper: mushroom, chard, kale, spinach, squash, asparagus, eggplant, green beans, potato, sweet potato, soybean, lentil, tomato, bell pepper.

Iodine: sea vegetables.

Iron: spinach, chard, lettuce, mushroom, green beans, parsley, kale, broccoli, Brussels sprout, asparagus, soybean, lentil, celery, cabbage.

Magnesium: most vegetables.

Manganese: green leafy vegetables, garlic, squash, beans, beets, peas, sea vegetables, bell pepper, celery, corn, cucumber, corn, endive, fennel, eggplant.

Molybdenum: bell pepper, celery, eggplant, lettuce, onion, tomato, green beans.

Phosphorus: most vegetables.

Potassium: most vegetables.

Selenium: asparagus, spinach, broccoli, garlic, mushroom, bamboo shoots, celery, mallow, sea vegetables, molokhia, parsnip.

Silicon: green beans, sea vegetables, samphire.

Sulphur: cauliflower, garlic, onion, parsnip, Brussels sprouts, celery, cucumber, mushroom, collard greens.

Zinc: mushroom, squash, green beans and peas, lettuce, parsley, arugula, asparagus, broccoli, endive, spinach, chard, collard greens.

Fibre: all vegetables.

Antioxidant flavonoids: most vegetables.

Tryptophan: mushroom, spinach, kale, asparagus, soybean, broccoli, cauliflower, chard, collard greens.

Omega-3 fatty acids: cauliflower, cabbage, lettuce, broccoli, Brussels sprout, squash, soybean, collard greens, spinach, kale, green beans.

Proteins: legumes, sea vegetables, mushroom, chard, asparagus, collard greens, cauliflower, broccoli.

ALZHEIMER'S DISEASE PROTECTORS

Oxidative damage caused by the amyloid peptides in the brain could be prevented by polyphenolic antioxidants present in some vegetables and fruits. The following vegetables have brain-boosting properties and the ability to defer the onset of dementia:

- Bok choy
- Mushroom
- Beets
- Squash
- Brussels sprout
- Beans
- Cabbage
- Celery
- Chard
- Collard greens
- Spinach
- Kale
- Parsley
- Endive
- Rhubarb
- Carrot

ANAEMIA CORRECTORS

Anaemia is a disorder that is caused by iron deficiency. Vegetables rich in iron and copper with vitamin C, which aid in the absorption of iron from the gut, correct this disorder:

- Asparagus
- Arugula
- Bok choy
- Chard
- Beets
- Spinach
- Dandelion greens
- Legumes
- Brussels sprout
- Kale
- Lettuce
- Kohlrabi
- Tomato
- Endive
- Broccoli

ANTI-AGEING AGENTS

Due to cumulative oxidative damage to the cells by free radicals, ageing, as shown by wrinkles, for example, occurs. Some vegetables slow down or even reverse the process of ageing:

- Asparagus
- Beets
- Carrot
- Collard
- Kale
- Molokhia
- Mustard greens
- Spinach
- Soybean
- Tomato

ANTI-ALLERGIC

Allergy is the immune system's reaction to certain environmental substances like pollen and ragweed. As a result of the interaction of allergens with immune cells, histamine is released in the bloodstream, causing allergic reactions like sneezing, wheezing, itchy eyes, and skin rash. The following vegetables, by virtue of their high content of quercetin, vitamin C, vitamin E, or omega-3 fatty acids, can help to reduce these symptoms:

- Onion
- Garlic
- Cayenne pepper
- Sweet potato
- Wasabi
- Mustard greens
- Broccoli
- Cauliflower
- Cucumber
- Carrot
- Celery
- Spinach
- Kale
- Lettuce
- Brussels sprout

ANTI-ARTHRITIC

Arthritis is a painful condition characterised by inflammation of joints, resulting in reduced mobility. Some vegetables lower the inflammation due to their antioxidant and anti-inflammatory properties and thus slow down the progress and severity of rheumatism:

+ Legumes
+ Brussels sprout
+ Carrot
+ Pumpkin
+ Broccoli
+ Sweet potato
+ Allium family (garlic, onion, leek, shallot, scallion, chives)
+ Chicory
+ Mustard greens
+ Horseradish
+ Celery
+ Collards
+ Squash
+ Artichoke
+ Molokhia
+ Kale
+ Dandelion greens
+ Spinach
+ Lettuce
+ Cucumber

On the other hand, members of the nightshade family, which grow during the night instead of the day (potatoes, tomatoes, eggplant), contain an alkaloid that triggers inflammation and worsens the severity of rheumatic symptoms.

Anti-Bleeding

Vitamin K is essential for the formation of prothrombin, a protein involved in the clotting process.

The following vegetables are involved in normal clot formation due to their high vitamin K content:

- Spinach
- Kale
- Brussels sprouts
- Asparagus
- Green onion
- Alfalfa sprouts
- Turnip greens
- Mustard greens
- Collard greens
- Chard
- Broccoli
- Cabbage
- Cauliflower
- Legumes

Patients taking thinning medications like warfarin and heparin, which inhibit clotting factors in the blood, prescribed to lower the risk of heart attack and stroke, should not eat large quantities of the above-mentioned vegetables to prevent bleeding more easily.

ANTI-CONSTIPATION

Constipation is passing hard dry stools with a frequency of less than three times per week. Low fibre diet, dehydration, sedentary lifestyle, certain diseases like hypothyroidism, and magnesium deficiency contribute to constipation.

Vegetables containing insoluble fibre add bulk to stool and stimulate the growth of good bacteria that help digestion. Digestive enzymes in some vegetables aid in relieving constipation. High water content of vegetables also assists in smooth bowel movement. Dark green leafy vegetables are also rich in magnesium, an important mineral involved in proper faecal elimination.

The following vegetables are useful in combating constipation:

+ Cabbage
+ Rhubarb
+ Legumes
+ Chlorophyll-rich vegetables like alfalfa, wheatgrass, and barley grass
+ Green leafy vegetables like spinach, kale, and chard
+ Chicory
+ Endive
+ Sweet potato
+ Squash
+ Carrot

ANTI-DIABETIC

Vegetarians have lower incidence of type 2 diabetes than non-vegetarians.

The following vegetables, due to their low caloric and carbohydrate content, their insulin-like effect on glucose metabolism, or high chromium content, or high fibre and antioxidant level, are ideal to be included in diabetic diets:

- Tubers (potatoes, leeks, yams)
- Legumes (beans, peas, lentils)
- Green leafy vegetables
- Mushrooms
- Garlic and onion
- Tomato
- Bitter gourd
- Okra
- Artichoke
- Chicory
- Asparagus
- Cucumber
- Squash
- Rhubarb
- Dandelion greens

ANTIDIARRHOEA

Diarrhoea is a loose watery stool occurring more than three times in one day. It can be caused by eating or drinking food contaminated by viruses, bacteria, parasites, or toxins, food allergies, side effect of medications such as antibiotics, intolerance to lactose in dairy products and intolerance to gluten in wheat products, or gastrointestinal diseases such as irritable syndrome.

Some vegetables like lettuce, mashed potato, and cooked carrot ease the symptoms of diarrhoea while others aggravate the severity of symptoms, which are as follows:

- Beets
- Broccoli
- Brussels sprouts
- Cabbage
- Cauliflower
- Corn
- Greens (collard, mustard, and turnip)

Anti-Flatulence

Flatulence is caused by gas in the bowel. Gas is a natural by-product of digestion. Most foods produce intestinal gas that cause bloating and discomfort.

Vegetables that produce excessive quantity of gas are rich in indigestible fibre, such as legumes, onion, cabbage, broccoli, cauliflower, Brussels sprouts, artichoke, asparagus, and carrot.

Constipation is also responsible for intestinal putrefaction that generates gas.

On the other hand, vegetables that prevent or decrease flatulence include the following:

- Fennel seeds
- Ginger
- Peppermint oil
- Basil
- Amaranth
- Lettuce
- Samphire
- Chayote

Anti-Hypertensive

High blood pressure is the major cause of several health ailments, such as heart attack, stroke, and kidney failure. Research has shown that switching to vegetarian diet lowers blood pressure.

The best vegetables to lower high blood pressure are those that are rich in potassium, magnesium, calcium, fibre, antioxidants, phytochemicals, and nitric oxide.

Vegetables having some of those nutrients include the following:

+ Celery
+ Garlic
+ Potato
+ Spinach
+ Soybean
+ Mushrooms
+ Carrot
+ Broccoli

ANTI-INFECTIVE

Some vegetables help prevent a variety of infections, including cold and flu, due to their high antioxidant properties:

- Allium family
- Tomato
- Broccoli
- Kale
- Spinach
- Cabbage
- Brussels sprout
- Radish
- Horseradish
- Parsnip
- Chard
- Dandelion greens

Probiotics are healthy bacteria found in fermented soybean products, sauerkraut, and pickles that promote gastrointestinal and immune health to prevent and cure some viral infections.

APHRODISIACS

Vegetarians have better sex life than non-vegetarians because they have less clogged arteries.

An aphrodisiac is a nutrient or substance that increases sexual desire (libido) and performance. Aphrodisiac is named after the goddess Aphrodite.

The following vegetables improve sex life by virtue of their effect on increasing blood flow, activating sex hormones, producing neurotransmitters that elevate mood or merely for psychological effect due to their phallic shape:

+ Arugula
+ Molokhia
+ Onion
+ Garlic
+ Horseradish
+ Ginger
+ Mustard
+ Asparagus
+ Carrot
+ Cucumber
+ Fennel
+ Tomato
+ Artichoke
+ Celery
+ Cauliflower
+ Mushrooms
+ Sea vegetables
+ Chilli peppers

Appetisers

Appetite is the desire for food. Appetisers are the best way to start the meal.

The following vegetables stimulate appetite:

- Parsley
- Onion
- Bell pepper
- Radish
- Daikon
- Wasabi
- Horseradish
- Celery
- Dandelion greens
- Chicory
- Fennel
- Endive

BONE BUILDERS

To build and maintain strong bones and to prevent osteoporosis (porous, easily breakable bones), we need some minerals (calcium, magnesium, phosphorus, potassium, zinc, boron, selenium, molybdenum, and manganese), and vitamins (D, C, B, and carotenoids) in our diet.

Research shows that vegetarians have a significantly lower rate of fracture than non-vegetarians.

The following vegetables are rich sources of nutrients involved in bone making:

- Asparagus
- Broccoli
- Bok Choy
- Cabbage
- Endive
- Arugula
- Brussels sprout
- Carrot
- Celery
- Corn
- Collard
- Leek
- Kohlrabi
- Okra
- Pumpkin
- Parsley
- Tomato
- Kale
- Squash

- Turnip
- Leek
- Green beans
- Green peas
- Lettuce
- Green onions

Some vegetables, like spinach and chard, contain oxalic acid that blocks calcium absorption from the gut.

BREAST-MILK FLOW ENHANCERS (GALACTOGOGUES)

Several vegetables and herbs are traditionally used by nursing mothers to stimulate milk production and secretion.

These nutrients increase milk supply by increasing prolactin to initiate the breast-milk let-down reflex or oxytocin to aid in milk ejection.

Vegetable and herbal galactogogues include the following:

- Fennel
- Luffa
- Rutabaga
- Alfalfa sprouts
- Barley grass
- Garlic
- Marshmallow roots
- Fenugreek
- Thistles
- Anise
- Coriander
- Dandelion
- Dill
- Nettle
- Red clover
- Vervain
- Raspberry
- Cumin
- Borage

CANCER FIGHTERS

Many types of cancers are diet-related. Most vegetables have the ability to inhibit cancer cell growth or reduce tumour sizes. They owe their cancer-fighting ability to their high content of fibre, antioxidants, and phytochemicals. Research has shown lower incidence of cancers in vegetarians.

Dark green leafy vegetables (lettuce, mustard green, chard, chicory, spinach, collard greens) contain carotenoids and fight against lung and breast cancers.

Cruciferous vegetables (broccoli, cauliflower, Brussels sprouts, cabbage, and kale) contain indoles and sulphoraphane, which fight against lung, stomach, colorectal, prostate, and bladder cancers.

Soy products contain phytoestrogens and genistein, which fight against breast and prostate cancers.

Allium family (garlic, onion, leeks, and chives) contain diallyl disulphide, which fights against skin, colon, and lung cancers.

Mushrooms contain lentinan, lectin, and thioproline, which fight against prostate and breast cancers.

Chilli peppers contain capsaicin, which fights against stomach cancer.

Tomato contains lycopene, which fights against prostate, breast, lung, stomach, and pancreatic cancers.

Carrot contains carotenes and falcarinol, which fight against lung, breast, bladder, prostate, and gastrointestinal cancers.

Sweet potato contains beta-carotene and polyphenols, which fight against colon, intestine, kidney, and prostate cancers.

Beans contain flavonoid antioxidants and fibre, which fight against prostate, breast, and digestive cancers.

Sea vegetables contain chlorophyllones, which fight against breast cancer.

CARDIOPROTECTORS

Heart diseases are the major causes of death in many countries. Food quality can influence heart diseases by either causing or preventing them.

Most vegetables due to their low content of saturated fats and calories and high content of dietary fibre, vitamins (folic acid, C, and E), minerals (potassium, magnesium, calcium, manganese, and selenium), omega-3 fatty acids, plant sterols, flavonoids, and nitrate that is converted in the body to the vasodilator nitric oxide, protect the body from heart diseases and heart attack. They achieve this by lowering the risk factors such as high blood pressure, high level of LDL, and high level of homocysteine (the dangerous amino acid that destroys blood vessels).

The following vegetables are among those having cardioprotective effects:

Green leafy vegetables (such as spinach, lettuce, Brussels sprouts, and broccoli)

- Cabbage family
- Garlic and onion
- Legumes
- Asparagus
- Tomato
- Carrot
- Bell pepper
- Squash
- Celery
- Beets
- Cucumber
- Sweet potato

- Sea vegetables
- Eggplant
- Fennel
- Rhubarb
- Parsley

DETOXIFIERS (TOXIN NEUTRALISERS)

Everyday, body accumulates toxic substances from food and air such as heavy metals, herbicides, pesticides and cleaning products that can cause chronic diseases and allergies.

The following vegetables assist in removing toxins and waste products from the body:

- Green leafy vegetables
- Garlic and onion
- Beets
- Sea vegetables
- Carrot
- Asparagus
- Broccoli
- Cucumber
- Sweet potato
- Cauliflower
- Artichoke
- Radish and horseradish
- Tomato
- Barley grass
- Wheat grass
- Endive
- Arugula

DIGESTIVE AID

The following vegetables contain soluble fibre and enzymes that aid in digestion:

- Carrot
- Squash
- Starchy tubers (potato, sweet potato, and yam)
- Turnip
- Rutabaga
- Parsley
- Parsnip
- Beets
- Cucumber
- Okra
- Fennel
- Dandelion greens
- Chicory
- Tomato
- Onion
- Fermented vegetables like sauerkraut and soy products

DIURETICS

A diuretic is a substance that aids in increasing urine output, thus flushing out excess fluid and toxins and lowering blood pressure.

The following vegetables are natural diuretics:

+ Asparagus
+ Artichoke
+ Beets
+ Brussels sprouts
+ Cabbage
+ Carrot
+ Celery
+ Cucumber
+ Dandelion greens
+ Endive
+ Fennel
+ Garlic
+ Horseradish
+ Lettuce
+ Onion
+ Parsley
+ Radish
+ Tomato
+ Watercress

Energy Boosters

All vegetables provide some calories, but the following vegetables are considered energy boosters because they increase blood sugar level quickly due to their easy digestion and absorption in the bloodstream:

- Beets
- Carrots
- Cassava
- Corn
- Malanga
- Potato
- Sweet potato
- Taro
- Water chestnut
- Yams

FAT BURNERS

Fat-burning vegetables are high in fibre and water but low in fat and calories. They add bulk to the diet, giving a feeling of fullness. Their high water content aids in flushing out fat from the body.

Some vegetables burn fat by spending more calories to digest than what they contain (negative energy balance). Raw vegetables are better fat burners than cooked vegetables because more energy is required to digest fibre in raw vegetables. Other vegetables function by increasing the metabolic rate and thus increasing energy expenditures.

Fat-burning vegetables include the following:

- Cruciferous vegetables such as broccoli, cabbage, cauliflower, and Brussels sprouts
- Green leafy vegetables such as kale, lettuce, and spinach
- Nightshade vegetables such as eggplant, peppers, and tomato
- Gourds such as cucumber and squash
- Root vegetables such as beets, carrots, celery, onion, radish, and turnip
- Legumes such as beans, peas, and lentils
- Mushrooms

HAIR CARE

Some vegetables can influence protecting some types of hair loss and greying. New hair growth can be stimulated by eating vegetables that contain hair-promoting nutrients such as vitamins (A, C, E, and biotin) and minerals (iron, calcium, zinc, and sulphur).

The following vegetables aid in hair care:

+ Sulphur-rich vegetables like garlic and onion
+ Sea vegetables rich in iodine
+ Legumes rich in protein, zinc, iron, and biotin
+ Peppers rich in vitamin C
+ Cruciferous vegetables like broccoli, cabbage, kale, cauliflower, and asparagus
+ Green leafy vegetables like spinach, chard, and lettuce rich in vitamins A and C
+ Carrot rich in vitamin A

HANGOVER OVER

Hangover is caused due to the poisonous amount of alcohol in the system, which produces hammering headache, nausea or vomiting, sweating, exhaustion, anxiety, and thirst. The main cause of thirst is dehydration caused by diuretic effect of alcohol, which increases urination. Alcohol also increases acidity, causing nausea and sweating. The cause of headache is dilatation of blood vessels in the head, pinching on the surrounding nerves.

The following vegetables reverse dehydration, restore the lost minerals, and detoxify the liver:

- Asparagus
- Bitter gourd
- Cucumber
- Artichoke
- Beetroot
- Celery
- Fennel
- Ginger

IMMUNITY BOOSTERS

Immune boosters increase white blood cells to fight infections and cancer.

Many nutrients such as vitamins (A, C, E, D, B6, and folic acid), minerals (zinc, selenium, manganese, iron, and copper), phytochemicals, and omega-3 fatty acids are involved in boosting immunity.

Daily consumption of five servings of the following vegetables boosts immunity:

- Cruciferous vegetables like broccoli, cauliflower, Brussels sprouts, and bok Choy
- Green leafy vegetables like spinach, chard, collard greens, and mustard greens
- Allium family like onion, garlic, chives, and leeks
- Orange vegetables like carrot, sweet potato, pumpkin, and winter squash
- Mushrooms

MIGRAINE PAIN

Migraine is a severe, pounding or pulsating headache on one side of the head accompanied by nausea or vomiting. It is caused by enlargement of blood vessels that cause the nerves to stretch, thus triggering the release of chemicals, which result in inflammation and pain.

The following vegetables ease migraine pain:

- The combination of carrot, spinach, beet, and cucumber juices
- Vegetables containing high vitamin B3 such as green leafy vegetables and tomato
- Vegetables containing high calcium and magnesium like green leafy vegetables
- Vegetables containing high level of vitamin B2 like broccoli, spinach, and soy
- Vegetables containing omega-3 fatty acids like soy and pumpkin seeds
- Vegetables containing tryptophan like black-eyed peas and pumpkin seeds

MOOD ELEVATORS

Tryptophan and vitamin B6 are needed for healthy nervous system and elevated mood. These two nutrients are involved in the synthesis of neurotransmitters such as serotonin needed for mood regulation, the hormone adrenaline that responds to stress, and GABA (gamma-aminobutyric acid) linked to relaxation.

Consumption of the following vegetables is associated with lifting up the mood and feeling of well-being with less fatigue, anxiety, irritability, sensitivity, or depression:

+ Garlic
+ Onion
+ Potato
+ Tomato
+ Green beans and green peas
+ Lettuce
+ Eggplant
+ Chicory
+ Beets

PREMENSTRUAL SYNDROME

Premenstrual syndrome (PMS) includes painful cramps in lower abdomen, fluid retention leading to bloating, breast engorgement and tenderness, vomiting, headache, muscle and joint pain, fatigue, insomnia, anxiety, depression, and mood swings.

Many nutrients such as fibre, which cleans up body's excess, oestrogen, calcium, magnesium, zinc, vitamins E, B1, and B6, and omega-3 fatty acids ease the symptoms of PMS.

Vegetables containing these nutrients or having a diuretic effect are useful in this regard.

The following vegetables are effective:

- Beans
- Asparagus
- Celery
- Dandelion greens
- Parsley
- Artichoke
- Watercress
- Rutabaga
- Fennel
- Cucumber

POSTMENOPAUSAL AIDS

Postmenopause means the period after a woman ceases having menses for twelve months after the last menstruation. It is associated with oestrogen deficiency and can cause hot flashes, vaginal dryness, urinary incontinence, urinary tract infection, joint pain, sleep disorder, mood swings, osteoporosis, and cardiovascular diseases.

Hormone replacement therapy (HRT) is effective in relieving some of these symptoms but could be associated with breast cancer, blood clots, stroke, or cardiovascular diseases.

Vegetables containing phytoestrogens (plant hormones) have some efficacy in easing postmenopausal symptoms in some women:

+ Soybean
+ Red clover
+ Rhubarb
+ Yam
+ Dandelion greens
+ Mustard

Pregnancy Ideals

During pregnancy, all nutrients are needed in higher amounts, especially protein (to increase muscle), iron (to increase blood volume), calcium (to form bone and storage for lactation), folic acid (to prevent neural tube defects like spina bifida), and fibre (to prevent haemorrhoids and constipation).

All vegetables are suitable during pregnancy but the following groups are ideal:

- Green leafy vegetables are rich in iron, folic acid, calcium, fibre, potassium, and vitamins A and C. They include spinach, cabbage, Brussels sprouts, celery, cauliflower, rhubarb, collard greens, and mustard greens.
- Yellow-orange vegetables like corn, pumpkin, and bell peppers contain a high amount of carotenoids and vitamin A.
- Roots and tubers like potato, sweet potato, carrot, yam, onion, garlic, turnip, radish, and rutabaga are rich in energy and potassium. Potassium maintains cardiac activity and blood pressure during pregnancy.
- High-fibre vegetables include asparagus, artichoke, broccoli, cucumber, eggplant, legumes, squash, mushrooms, okra, and bell pepper.
- Some vegetables like bitter gourd are beneficial in gestational diabetes.

SINUS RELIEVERS

Sinusitis is the inflammation of sinuses and nasal passages caused by interference with airflow into sinuses, blocking mucous drainage.

Major causes of sinusitis are infections, polyps, and allergies.

Sinusitis causes headache, nasal stuffiness, facial pain, cough, and fever.

Vegetables containing vitamin A, vitamin C, and omega-3 fatty acids are effective in relieving the symptoms of sinusitis. Other vegetables with pungent flavour are also effective in this regard:

- Garlic
- Onion
- Daikon
- Wasabi
- Radish
- Horseradish
- Luffa
- Juice made of carrot, cucumber, and beet

Skin Care

Antioxidants, zinc and vitamins C, E, and A, prevent wrinkles, puffiness, and dryness, creating glowing skin.

Vegetables that have skin-beautifying properties include the following:

- Tomato
- Potato
- Sweet potato
- Molokhia
- Pumpkin
- Spinach
- Soybean
- Sea vegetables
- Cucumber
- Radish
- Horseradish
- Kale
- Collard greens
- Asparagus
- Broccoli
- Cauliflower

SLEEPING AID

Nutrients that induce sleep include the following:

- Tryptophan, the amino acid that helps the body make serotonin, which slows down nerve impulses and promotes calm and is the precursor of melatonin
- Melatonin, which regulates sleep cycles
- Vitamin B6 needed to make serotonin
- Carbohydrates, which raise blood insulin level, which helps the tryptophan in the blood to enter the brain and produce high level of serotonin
- Magnesium, which relaxes muscle spasm

Vegetables rich in these nutrients include the following:

- Green leafy vegetables like kale, chard, and spinach
- Chickpeas (hummus)
- Potato
- Celery
- Lettuce
- Beets
- Squash
- Purslane
- Asparagus
- Beans and soy

Avoid spicy vegetables like garlic, hot pepper, and ginger before sleep

Many fruits also induce sleep like apple, banana, tart cherries, grapes, red dates, guava, and kiwi.

Have sweet dreams.

STROKE PREVENTERS

Many factors such as high blood pressure, cardiovascular diseases, diabetes, high cholesterol, high homocysteine, and high fibrinogen levels in the blood increase the risk of ischemic stroke.

Research has shown that increased consumption of vegetables, fruits, whole grains, and fish rich in omega-3 fatty acids reduce the risk of stroke.

Vegetables rich in fibre, folic acid, vitamin B6, potassium, omega-3 fatty acids, and phytochemicals have protective effect against stroke.

Such vegetables include the following:

+ Kale
+ Greens (turnip, mustard, collard)
+ Spinach
+ Chard
+ Broccoli
+ Cabbage
+ Lettuce
+ Cauliflower
+ Brussels sprouts
+ Bok choy
+ Parsley
+ Carrot
+ Pumpkin
+ Celery
+ Garlic, onion, and leeks
+ Sea vegetables

ULCER HEALER

Gastritis, the inflammation of gastric lining, is mainly caused by drugs or by the bacterium H. pylori. If it is untreated, it could lead to peptic ulcer, and that in turn could cause stomach cancer.

Vegetables containing high fibre, Vitamin A, vitamin C, vitamin E, zinc, and flavonoids help in re-establishing healthy gastrointestinal lining and thus healing the ulcer.

The following vegetables have been shown to have ulcer-healing properties:

- Cabbage juice
- Broccoli
- Cauliflower
- Cucumber
- Sweet potato
- Turnips
- Bell pepper
- Bitter gourd
- Carrot
- Soy
- Green beans
- Green peas
- Squash
- Celery

Avoid tomato-based products, chilli pepper, citrus fruits, coffee, tea, alcohol, sodas, and most importantly stress.

Vision Enhancers

Vegetables rich in antioxidant vitamins (A, C, and E), carotenoids (beta-carotene, lycopene, lutein, and zeaxanthin), omega-3 fatty acids, and zinc delay the onset of age-related macular degeneration and cataract and prevent night blindness.

The following vegetables have vision-enhancing properties:

+ Green leafy vegetables such as spinach and kale
+ Yellow-orange vegetables like carrot, sweet potato, corn, and pumpkin
+ Red vegetables like tomato and beets
+ Bell peppers
+ Soy, green beans, and green peas
+ Sulphur-containing vegetables like garlic and onion that improve blood vessels around the eyes

WEIGHT GAIN

The most important factor in gaining weight is to get energy surplus, which means consuming more calories than energy expenditure. The excess energy will be deposited by the body as fat or glycogen.

To gain weight on vegetables is not an easy job because vegetables have high content of water and fibre and low content of fat and protein.

To gain weight on vegetables, include several servings of starchy vegetables:

- Potato
- Sweet potato
- Corn
- Beetroot
- Carrot
- Malanga
- Cassava
- Yams
- Taro
- Water chestnut
- Protein-rich foods like legumes
- Soy

To add more calories to your vegetables, the following actions are beneficial:

- Eating creamy vegetable soups rather than clear soups
- Topping vegetables with butter, sauces, cheese, or gravy
- Adding nuts, seeds, or dried fruits to your salad
- Avoiding water-rich vegetables like cucumber, zucchini, broccoli, and cauliflower

WEIGHT LOSS

Losing weight by vegetables is much easier than gaining weight by them because most vegetables are rich in fibre and water but low in calories, fat, and protein. To lose weight, one must create a negative energy balance, which means spending more energy than caloric intake.

All dieting regimens include multiple daily servings of non-starchy vegetables with high content of fibre. High fibre increases basal metabolic rate (BMR) and makes the person feel full longer, resulting in less eating.

High fibre and high water content vegetables include the following:

- Brussels sprouts
- Asparagus
- Broccoli
- Cauliflower
- Spinach
- Endive
- Celery
- Rhubarb
- Tomato
- Bell peppers
- Cucumber
- Mushrooms

Garlic, ginger, and chilli peppers increase body temperature and boost metabolism.

Diuretic vegetables like artichoke, dandelion greens, fennel, parsley, radish, horseradish, and onion assist in lowering body weight by getting rid of excess fluid and salt.

Avoid starchy vegetables like potato, sweet potato, corn, beetroots, and carrot.

Substitute creamy vegetable soups with clear broth.

Avoid adding butter, sauces, oils, or cheese to your vegetables.

WHEEZING CEASING

Asthma is caused by inflammation in the bronchial tubes of lungs and contraction of the muscles surrounding them, which leads to mucous production that narrows airway passages, causing shortness of breath, wheezing, cough, and chest tightness.

Factors that trigger asthma attacks are pollens, mites, dust, smog, etc.

Emergency treatment of asthma attacks involves the use of bronchodilators and steroids.

Some vegetables, due to anti-inflammatory effect of their antioxidants and omega-3 fatty acids, lower the risk and severity of asthma.

Vegetables that are beneficial in asthma prevention and treatment include the following:

- Artichoke
- Asparagus
- Cauliflower
- Kale
- Molokhia
- Mustard greens
- Radish
- Horseradish
- Dandelion greens
- Garlic
- Onion
- Carrot

- Fennel
- Pumpkin
- Parsley
- Sweet potato

Avoid nightshade vegetables that trigger asthma such as tomato, peppers, eggplant, and potato.

This book, *The Miracle of Vegetables*, is intended to make the readers of all ages know the benefits of including several servings of vegetables in their daily diets. Furthermore, it describes common and rare vegetables consumed throughout the world and highlights their nutritional values and medicinal properties. The readers will come to learn which vegetables to select to prevent ailments like cancers, obesity, heart diseases, stroke, asthma, arthritis, Alzheimer's, depression, insomnia, indigestion, anorexia, menstrual problems, birth defects, allergies, anaemia, migraine, hangover, fatigue, and haemorrhoids; how to take care of skin, hair, liver, and eye; and how to boost immunity and libido.

AUTHOR

Dr Bahram Tadayyon, MNS, MD, Ph.D., from the Kingdom of Bahrain, is an internationally renowned nutritionist, who, besides his medical degree, has obtained his master's degree and doctorate in nutrition from Cornell University in New York. He has taught nutrition to medical students in several countries and has written several books related to nutrition. His last book *The Miracle of Fruits* was well received by the professionals in medical fields and by those who have interest in alternative, natural way to heal diseases.